Pregnancy

A

Beginners Guide to

Pregnancy, Childbirth, Breastfeeding

and Circumcision

By

Dr. Jane Smart

www.MillenniumPublishingLimited.com

Copyright 2018

All rights reserved. This document is geared towards providing exact and reliable information in regards to the topic and issue covered. The publication is sold on the idea that the publisher is not required to render an accounting, officially permitted, or otherwise, qualified services. If advice is necessary, legal or professional, a practiced individual in the profession should be ordered.

In no way is it legal to reproduce, duplicate, or transmit any part of this document by either electronic means or in printed format. Recording of this publication is strictly prohibited, and any storage of this document is not allowed unless with written permission from the publisher. All rights reserved.

The information provided herein is stated to be truthful and consistent, in that any liability, regarding inattention or otherwise, by any usage or abuse of any policies, processes, or directions contained within is the solitary and utter responsibility of the recipient reader. Under no circumstances will any legal responsibility or blame be held against the publisher for any reparation, damages, or monetary loss due to the information herein, either directly or indirectly. Respective authors own all copyrights not held by the publisher. The information herein is offered for informational purposes solely and is universal as so. The presentation of the information is without a contract or any guarantee assurance.

The trademarks that are used are without any consent, and the publication of the mark is without permission or backing by the trademark owner. All trademarks and brands within this book are for clarifying purposes only and are owned by the owners themselves, not affiliated with this document.

Download For FREE

If you want to download a booklet that summarizes more than 45 frequently asked questions about pregnancy then you are in luck! A PDF version of the below book is located at a certain place and can be downloaded for FREE. However, a password is required to unlock the download. Follow the steps below to retrieve the password!

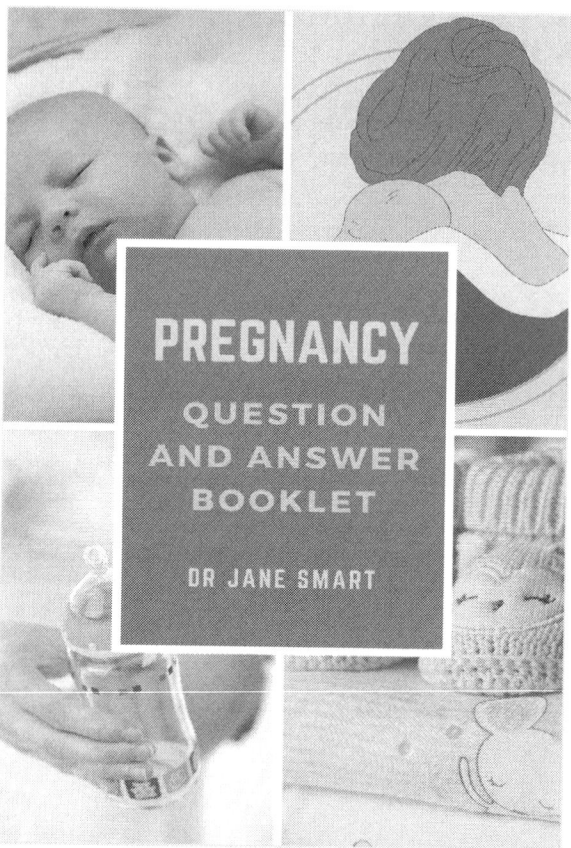

Steps to take

1. The password consists of 6 characters (all lower case)
2. Here is the incomplete password: -a-g-s

3. The first, third and fifth character of the password is missing and is located in random pages of this book.

4. Read this book carefully to locate and retrieve them (they're so obvious you can't miss them).

5. Once you have the complete password then click the below Enter Password button or go to www.MillenniumPublishingLimited.com > Dr. Jane Smart > Pregnancy Q&A Booklet, enter the password, download the booklet and enjoy!

-a-g-s

Enter Password

Table of Contents

Part 1 – Pregnancy and Childbirth

Introduction 16

Chapter 1 20
- **Early Pregnancy Symptoms** 20
  - a) A missed period: 20
  - b) Fatigue: 21
  - c) Abdominal bloating: 21
  - d) A frequent need to urinate: 21
  - e) Food aversion: 22
  - f) Sore breasts: 22
  - g) Mood swings: 22
  - h) Elevated basal temperature: 22
  - i) Spotting: 23
  - j) Nausea and/or vomiting: 23

Chapter 2 25
- **Pregnancy Test** 25
  - When is the right time to take a pregnancy test? 25

Chapter 3 28
- **Pregnancy Due Date** 28

Chapter 4 30
- **Antenatal Screening** 30
  - What can an ultrasound scan determine? 31
  - What blood tests will you have? 32

Chapter 5 36
- **Nutrition in Pregnancy** 36
  - a) Fruits and vegetables: 37
  - b) Protein: 38
  - c) Carbohydrates (starchy foods): 39
  - d) Dairy Foods: 40
  - e) Iron: 41
- **What foods should I avoid during pregnancy?** 42
  - a) Certain cheese: 43
  - b) Cream and custard: 43
  - c) Hummus: 43

  d) Pate: 43
  e) Raw or partially cooked eggs: 43
  f) Raw, cured and undercooked meat: 44
  g) Liver: 44
  h) Some types of fish: 44
  i) Raw shellfish: 44
  j) Pre-prepared chilled meals and leftovers: 45
  k) Caffeine: 45
  l) Sushi: 46

Chapter 6 48
Weight Gain and Exercise During Pregnancy 48
  Bikram yoga (Hot yoga): 50
  Horse riding, gymnastics and cycling: 50
  Contact sports: 51
  Scuba diving: 51
Other do's and don'ts 51
Postnatally 51

Chapter 7 53
Embryo and Foetal Development 53
  Week 3: 53
  Weeks 4 to 5: 54
  Week 6: 54
  Week 8: 54
  Week 10: 55
  Week 12: 55
  Weeks 13 to 16: 55
  Weeks 17 to 20: 56
  Weeks 21 to 24: 56
  Week 25 to 28: 57
  Weeks 29 to 32: 57
  Weeks 33 to 36: 58
  Weeks 37 to 40: 58

Chapter 8 60
Changes During Pregnancy 60
  Respiratory System 60
  Cardiovascular System 60
  Gastrointestinal System 60

    Endocrine System 61
    Uterus 61
    Urinary System 62
    Musculoskeletal System 62
    Skin 62
    Spider veins 62
    Varicose vein 63
    Stretch marks 63
    Breasts 63
    Other changes 64

Chapter 9 65
Pregnancy Trimesters 65
    First Trimester 65
    Second Trimester 66
    Third Trimester 66

Chapter 10 69
Sex During Pregnancy 69

Chapter 11 71
High Risk Pregnancy 71
    Smoking Complications: 72
    Alcohol: 72
    Hyperemesis Gravidarum (HG): 73
    Gestational Diabetes: 74
    Pre-eclampsia: 74
    Ectopic Pregnancy: 75
    Placenta Previa: 75
    Placental Abruption: 76
    Premature Labour: 76
Social Factors 77
    Older mums 77
    Teen Pregnancy 78
    Bed Rest 79

Chapter 12 80
What Do I Need to Take Into Hospital? 80
    Home Equipment Considerations 82

Refresher 87

Pregnancy Q & A's 87

Conclusion 113

Part II - Breastfeeding, Diapering and Circumcision

Introduction II 117

Chapter 13 119
History of Infant Feeding 119

Chapter 14 123
Historical Alternatives to Breastfeeding 123

Chapter 15 124
Social Pressure & infant Feeding 124

Chapter 16 126
Breastfeeding Basics 126

Chapter 17 132
Contraindication to Breastfeeding 132

Chapter 18 135
Exclusive Pumping 135

Chapter 19 139
Donor Breast Milk 139

Chapter 20 140
Bottle-feeding 140
Breastfeeding Positions 142

Chapter 21 152
Breastfeeding Diet 152
Snacks for the Breastfeeding Mother 152
Supplementation 153
Breastfeeding Tips 154

Chapter 22 155
Frequently Asked Questions 155

Chapter 23 168
Myths and Misperceptions 168

Chapter 24 176

Breastfeeding Accessories 176
- 1. Breastfeeding pillow 176
- 2. Breast pads 176
- 3. Milk-saver 177
- 4. Breast pump 177
- 5. Pumping bra 178
- 6. Breastfeeding bottles 178
- 7. Breastfeeding cover 178
- 8. Breast Milk Storage Bags 179
- 9. Breastfeeding Bras 179
- 10. Breastfeeding Clothing 179
- 11. Lanolin Cream 180
- 12. Gel Pads 180
- 13. Cold Packs 180
- 14. Nipple Everter 181
- 15. Breast Shells 181
- 16. Nipple Shield 181
- 17. Breast Milk Alcohol Test Strips 182

Chapter 25 183
Bathing Techniques 183
- Types of Baby Bathtubs 189
- Basic Baby Bathing Tips 194

Chapter 26 199
Baby Diapering Methods 199
- A. Cloth Diapering 200
- B. Disposable Diapers 200
- Comparison between both types 201
- Cloth Diaper Considerations 202
- Types of Cloth Diapers 204
- More on Disposable Diapering 207
- Diapering Tips 207

Chapter 27 211
Baby Circumcision 211
- Care of the intact penis 212
- The Great Circumcision Debate 214
- Risks Associated with Circumcision 215
- The Circumcision Procedure 215

    After the Circumcision 216
    Female circumcision 218
    Female Genital Mutilation as a Social Norm 219
    Why FGM is Performed 220
    Anatomy of Female genitalia 221
    Morality of FGM 223
    Legality of FGM 223
    International Outcry 226

Follow me **228**

References **235**

This Bundle Consist of:

Pregnancy – The Ultimate Guide to Pregnancy and Childbirth (Part I)

Breastfeeding – A Beginners Guide to Infant Feeding, Diapering and Circumcision (Part II)

Part I

Pregnancy

The

Ultimate Survival Guide to

Pregnancy and Birth

By

Dr. Jane Smart

www.MillenniumPublishingLimited.com

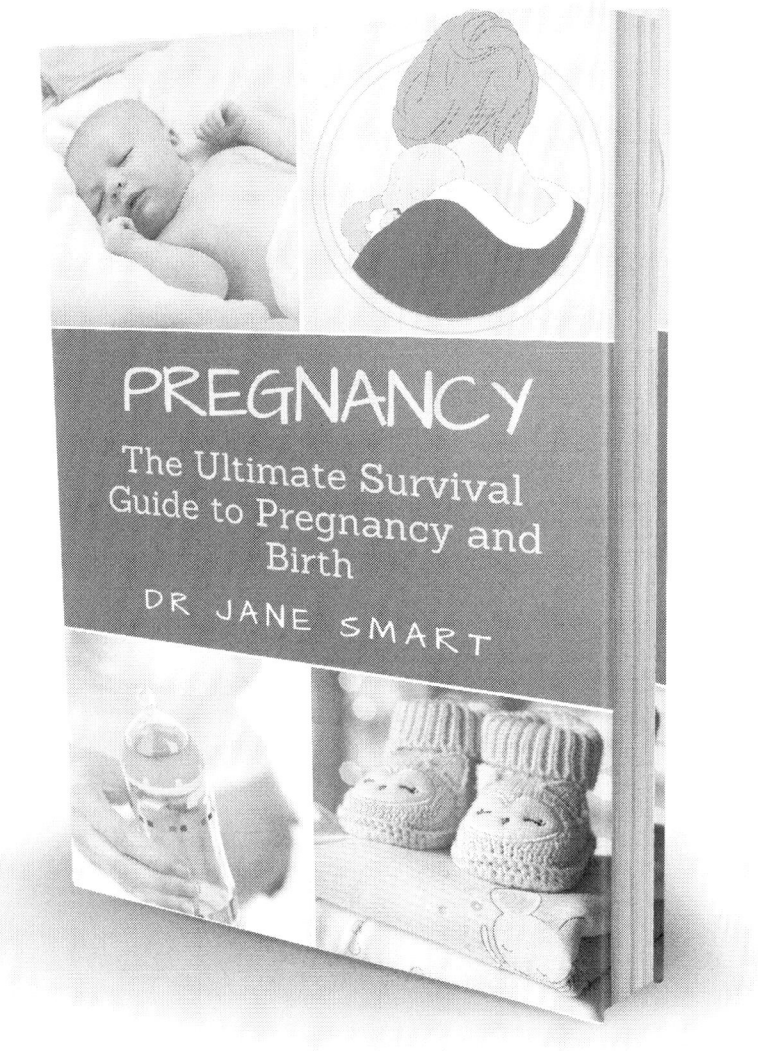

Available in kindle, Paperback and Audio format

Introduction

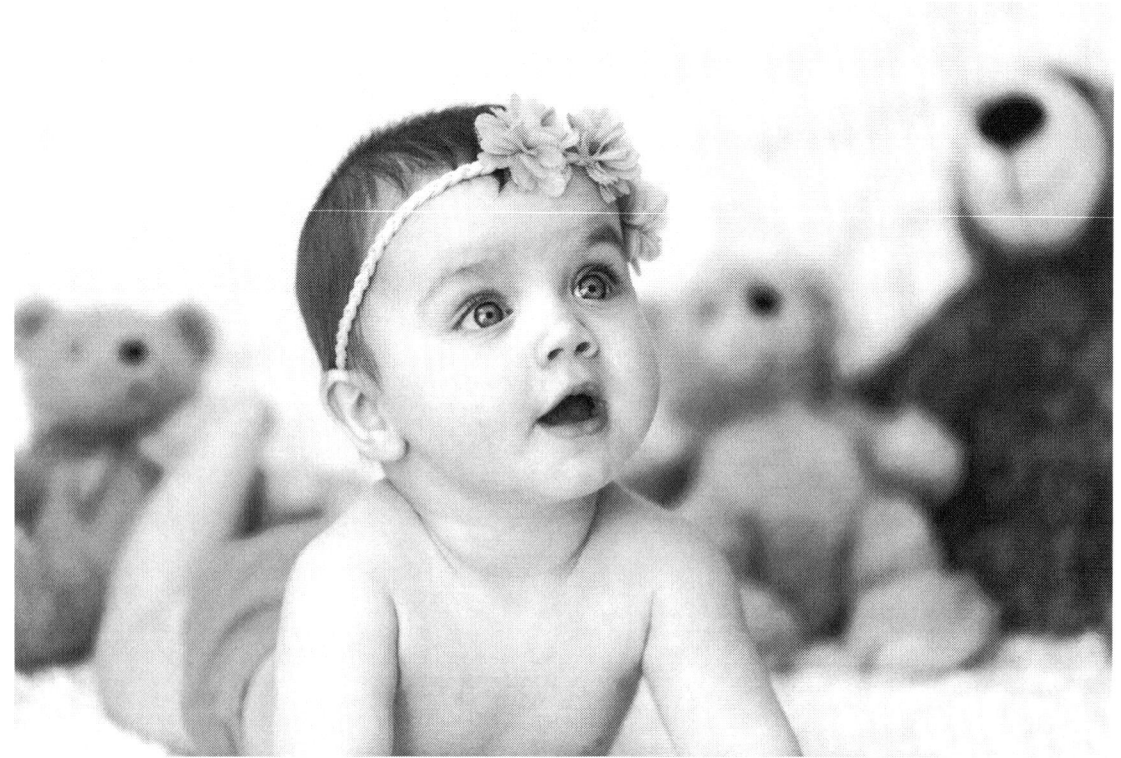

Congratulations, you're pregnant! In approximately nine-month's-time a baby boy or girl will arrive in your life, and the real responsibility begins. Rest assured, this book is aimed at helping you cope: Look upon it as your pregnancy companion. We cover topics from trimesters of pregnancy (pregnancy stages), prenatal care, to dietary do's and don'ts.

There is a lot to contend with whilst pregnant and it helps to be prepared. This book is aimed at all mums-to-be. No two pregnancies are the same, and some may have issues to overcome e.g. nausea and vomiting, so it can be useful to have helpful information to hand. Pregnancy is an exciting journey and you are probably more prepared than you realise. If not, this book will provide you with facts around 'what to expect when you are expecting'.

The terms pregnant and prenatal are derived from the Latin words pre - meaning before, and (g)natus - meaning birth. Therefore 'before gives birth'. You may also hear health professionals use the term gestation. This is the period or process, from conception to birth, of the baby developing in the womb.

Pregnancy officially starts from the first day of a woman's last normal menstrual period, even though the development of the fetus does not begin until conception, which is two weeks later. This is because every time you have a period your body is preparing for pregnancy. It also serves as a gauge for health professionals, as it is difficult for them to know precisely when conception occurred. Your expected delivery date is therefore calculated 40 weeks and from the first day of your last period.

Pregnancy consists of three trimesters: First, second and third, which are roughly three months in duration. For the first 10 weeks of your pregnancy (or 8 weeks after conception) your baby is referred to as an embryo. From 10-weeks onwards your baby is known as a foetus. A baby is considered full term from the beginning of the 39th to the end of the 40th week of pregnancy. Typically, a woman will give birth between her 39th and 42nd week, when the pregnancy is left to progress naturally.

Please note: this book is in no way a replacement for the professional care a midwife or doctor can provide. So please talk to them if anything is concerning you

Congratulations!

The first character of the password required to unlock the Pregnancy Question & Answer booklet is letter n.

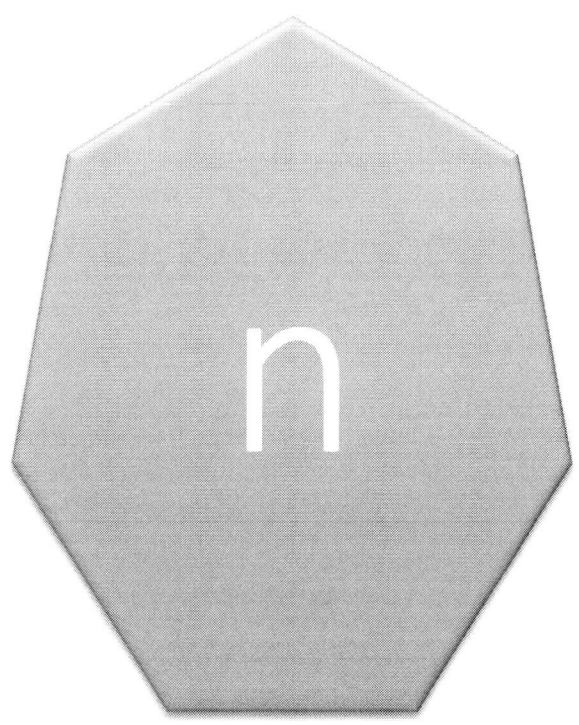

Chapter 1

Early Pregnancy Symptoms

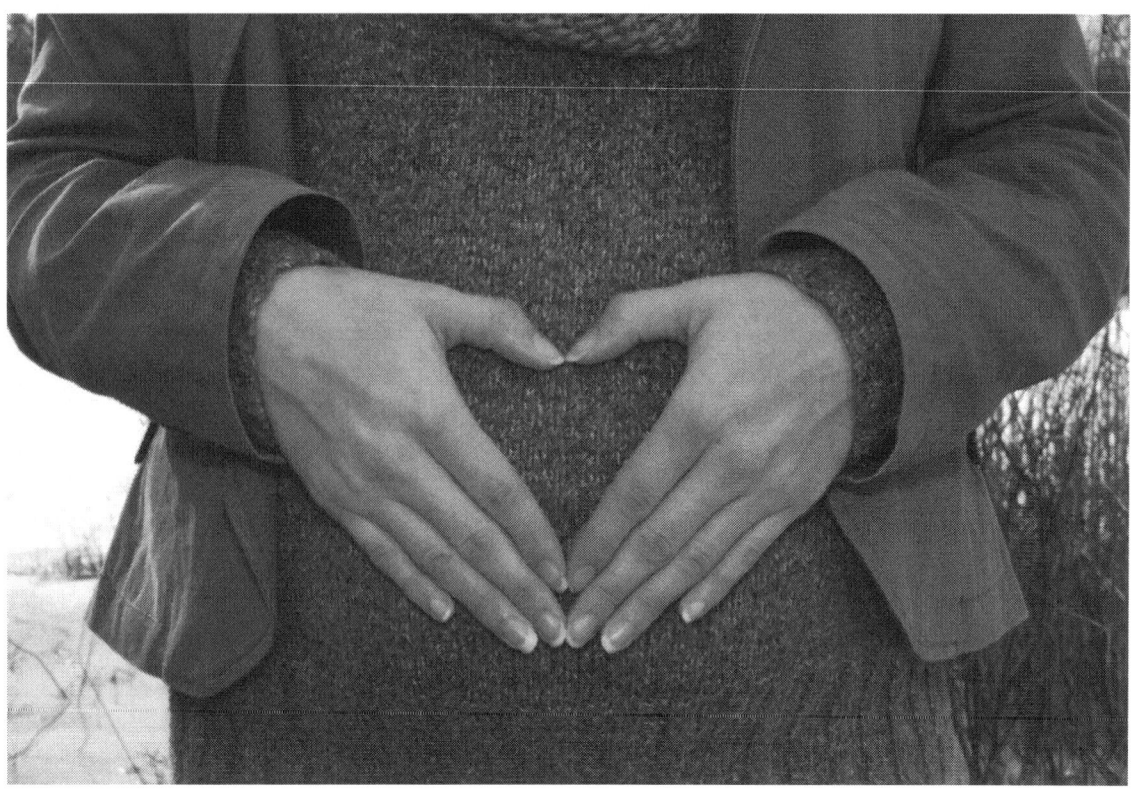

There are a variety of symptoms you may experience during early pregnancy. Not all women experience the same ones, and they can differ with successive pregnancies. Some can appear when you have missed a period, others not for a few weeks. Here are a few:

a) A missed period:

Women that have regular periods, but then miss one may do a pregnancy test before any other symptoms occur. For others with irregular periods, the first inkling they might be pregnant could be breast tenderness, nausea or needing the loo more often!

b) Fatigue:

You might not just feel sleepy, you may be exhausted! Although no one is sure, it may be the increase of the hormone progesterone that makes you feel tired. Obviously, if you need to wee more often and you feel sick, this can add to the tiredness. Women usually start to have more energy once into the 2nd trimester. Tiredness will usually return in late pregnancy, when the weight of the baby can make it harder for you to get a good night's sleep. Be sure to rest when the chance arises and accept help if it is offered. Remember housework can wait, looking after yourself comes first!

c) Abdominal bloating:

As with a period, the hormones associated with early pregnancy can make you feel bloated. So even though there is no outward sign of pregnancy your clothes may feel a little tight.

d) A frequent need to urinate:

Hormonal changes in pregnancy mean that the blood flow to your kidneys increases. This means your bladder fills more quickly, which in turn makes you urinate more often! This frequent need to wee increases later in pregnancy, when the baby's weight puts more pressure on your bladder.

e) Food aversion:

It can be common for women in early pregnancy to feel nauseated when confronted with certain smells e.g. coffee, spicy food. It can often be things that you really enjoyed prior to pregnancy. Strong smells may even make you want to gag. Although experts do not know for certain why this occurs, it may be due to the increasing amount of oestrogen in your system.

f) Sore breasts:

Rising hormone levels can cause sensitive swollen breasts, again like before a period. This should ease after your first trimester, as your body becomes more used to the hormonal changes

g) Mood swings:

These are common in early pregnancy, and are due to hormone changes that effect the chemical messengers in your brain. Some mums-to-be may feel a positive effect, others may feel depressed or anxious. If you are finding it hard to cope, make sure to contact your healthcare provider immediately.

h) Elevated basal temperature:

Your basal temperature is the lowest measurement of your body's temperature, when taken first thing in the morning. Some women chart their temperature, to establish when they are due to ovulate, and therefore more likely to conceive. If it remains high for over 2 weeks, then you are likely pregnant.

i) Spotting:

It is natural to feel concerned, if after wanting to be pregnant, you then see bleeding. If this happens around the time you would normally have a period, it could be due to implantation bleeding, i.e. the fertilized egg settling in the lining of your womb. If the bleeding is severe, accompanied by pain, or you just need reassurance, contact your midwife or doctor.

j) Nausea and/or vomiting:

Commonly known as 'morning sickness'. It usually starts at about 8 weeks into pregnancy, but for some women it can appear as early as 2 weeks. It can also occur any time of day or night. Nausea will normally begin to ease by the start of the 2nd trimester. Some of the following may mean you are at more risk of developing nausea and vomiting.

- A first pregnancy.
- Multiple pregnancy e.g. twins or triplets.
- Nausea and vomiting in a previous pregnancy.
- A family history of nausea and vomiting in pregnancy. For example, if your mum experienced morning sickness carrying you, you may find you will too!
- If you have experienced nausea when using contraceptives that contain oestrogen.
- If you suffer from motion sickness: for example, travelling in a car.
- Being obese, with a body mass index (BMI) of 30 or more.

- Stress.

We cover what you can do to help nausea and vomiting in the Q & A section at the end of this book.

Chapter 2

Pregnancy Test

Many home pregnancy tests are not sensitive enough to detect you are pregnant until approximately a week after you've missed a period. If it shows a negative result, wait a few days and try again. Looking after your health is vital, even if you don't have a positive result yet.

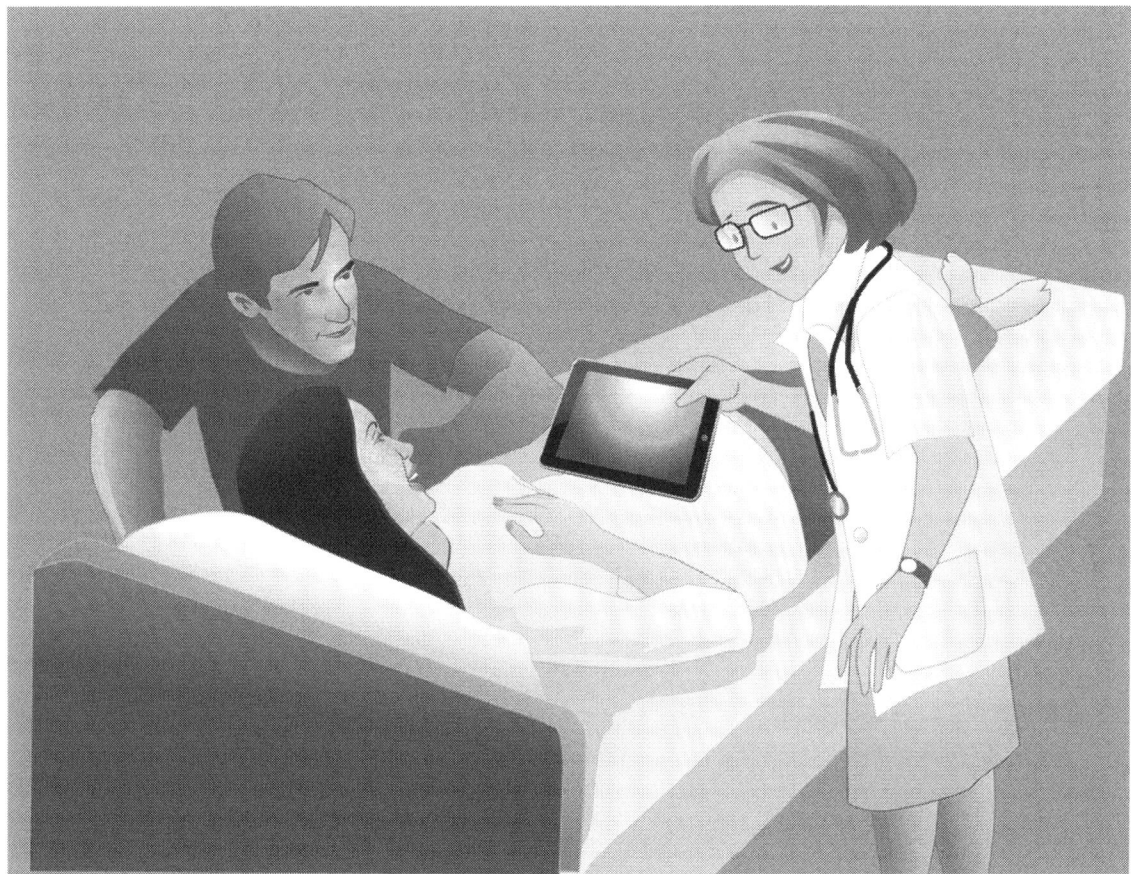

When is the right time to take a pregnancy test?

There are different pregnancy tests available, depending on the timing of conception and your preference; There is the classic urine test and a blood test.

The hormone present in your body during pregnancy is called human chorionic gonadotrophin (hCG). It is produced by the placenta shortly after the embryo attaches to the wall of the uterus, and can usually be detected in urine six to twelve days after the egg has been fertilized. The hCG produced doubles every two to three days.

It is advisable to wait until the first day of your missed period to take a pregnancy test. This ensures that the level of hCG is high enough to be detected. It is recommended you take a pregnancy test using the first urine of the day, due to the urine being more concentrated, therefore the hCG level is easier to detect.

A blood test can be taken by your midwife or doctor. It also detects the presence of the hormone, hCG and can be performed six to eight days after ovulation. There are two types of blood tests: Qualitative and quantitative. A qualitative test gives a simple yes or no answer to whether you are pregnant or not. The quantitative tests, also known as beta hCG, shows the exact level of hormone found in your blood.

If you think you are pregnant but received a negative result with your home pregnancy test, don't worry. False-negatives can occur due to a variety of factors: The urine was too dilute to detect hCG; the test was done incorrectly or you tested too soon, or home pregnancy test has passed its use by date. Fertility medication, or other drugs containing hCG can interfere with home pregnancy tests. However, other medications, such as antibiotics or birth control pills shouldn't.

It is rare, but false-positives do occur and can be due to blood or protein being present in your urine. Certain drugs, such as anticonvulsants or tranquilisers can also cause false-positive test results.

Whether you have received a positive or negative result with a home pregnancy test, it is always best to seek the advice of a medical professional as soon as possible.

Chapter 3

Pregnancy Due Date

How can you calculate your baby's due date? Women do not have identical menstrual cycles; and if you have irregular periods your due date may be difficult to pinpoint. However, if you have a regular menstrual cycle of 28 days, you can estimate a due date by adding 280 days (9 months, 7 days) to the first day of your last period. Please remember this is not always 100% accurate and should be taken as an estimate only.

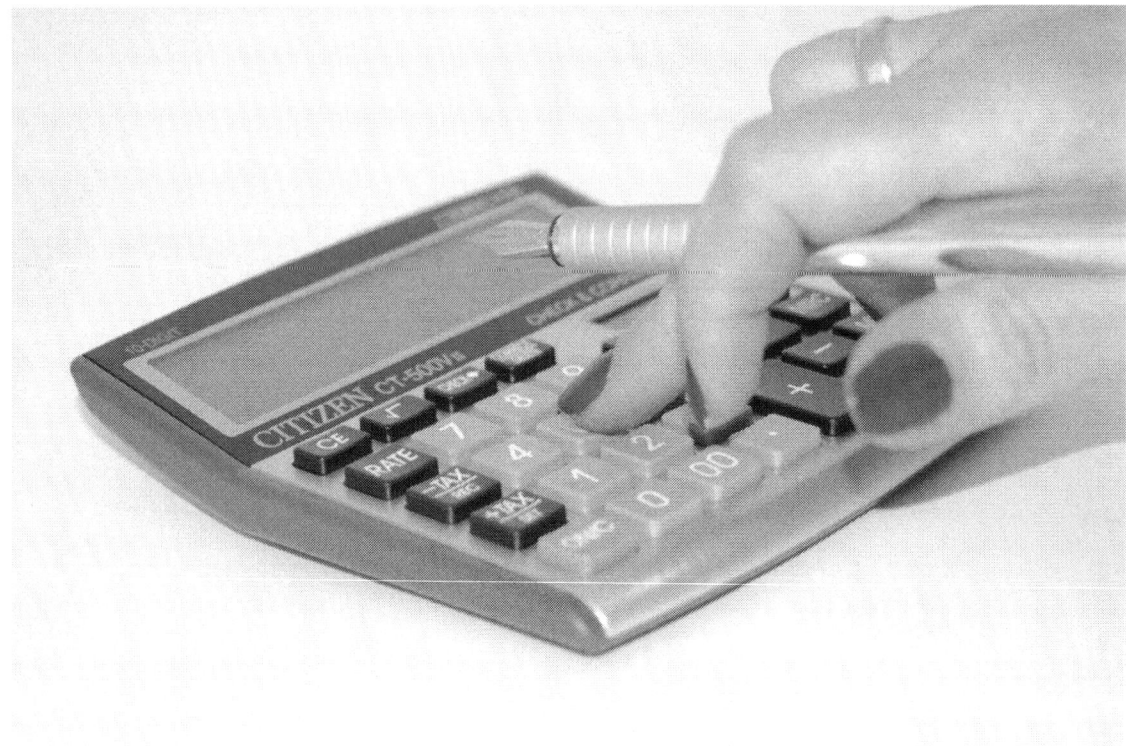

Your last menstrual period and ovulation are included in the first two weeks of your pregnancy. This may seem strange, as it means you are officially pregnant before you conceive! Only 5% of babies are born on their due date. 80% of women deliver somewhere between 37 and 42 weeks, which means approximately 15% deliver prematurely. Although there may not always be an obvious reason, there are certain risk factors that mean you may go into labour early e.g. multiple pregnancy, infection.

If you are a woman that has irregular periods, how can you determine your due date? First, if you can remember the date of your last menstrual cycle you can still use the calculation above. Another way for a midwife to estimate your baby's due date is to palpate your abdomen. They assess the fundal height: this is the top of the uterus (which reaches your navel at around 20 weeks.) An ultrasound scan can also be performed to determine your expected due date, if other methods have not worked or your midwife wants to confirm it.

A caesarean section is an alternate way to give birth and your due date may not be the only thing to consider, if one is required. They are usually scheduled no sooner than 7 days before your due date.

However, and whenever your baby is born, enjoy the moment. Many women would tell you, babies usually come when they are ready, and remember a due date is just an estimate!

Chapter 4

Antenatal Screening

Screening is an important part of pregnancy. When to test and what tests to have are important questions; and whether you are pregnant with your first child or been pregnant before, any testing can be nerve-wracking. Antenatal screening is carried out in all three trimesters. Each test is important, as they help assess both you and your baby's health, at different stages of your journey.

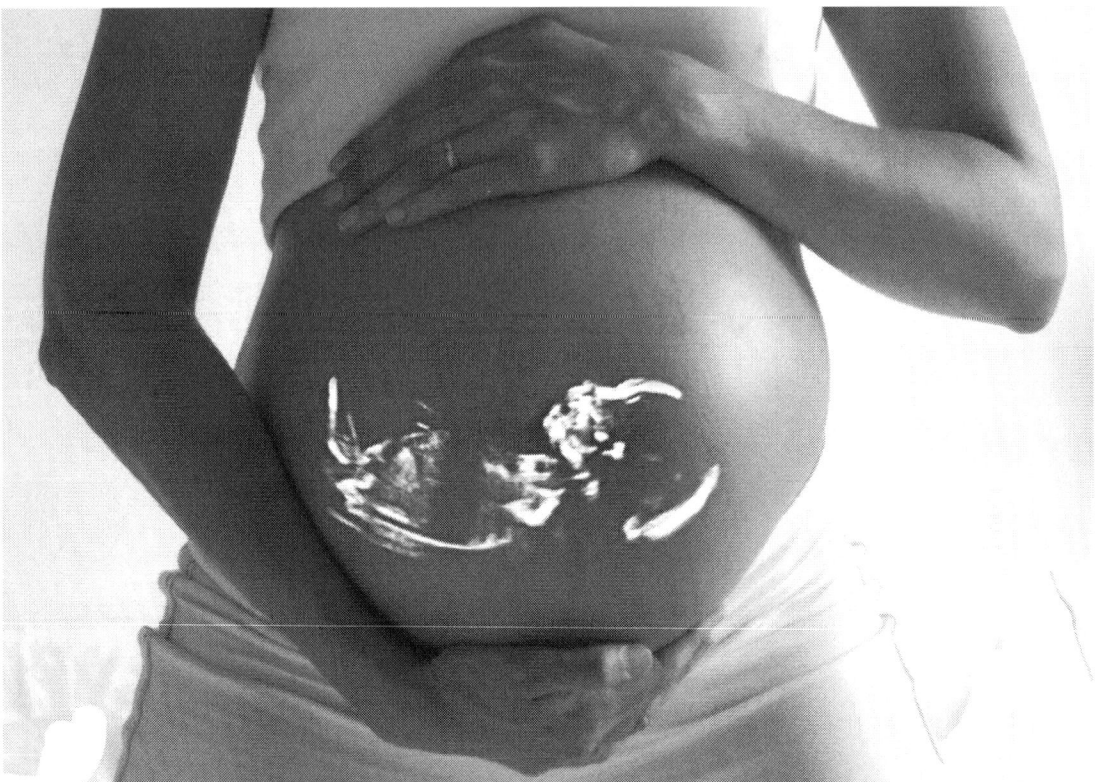

Hospitals in the UK offer all pregnant women at least two ultrasound scans during pregnancy. There are no known risks to either you or your baby, but it is important to make sure you have all the facts before having an ultrasound. If you choose not to go ahead, your choice will be respected, and you can continue with all other aspects of antenatal screening. Talk to you midwife/doctor about your concerns.

What can an ultrasound scan determine?
- Your baby's size. The dating scan will give you a better idea of how many weeks pregnant you are.
- Whether you are having one, or more babies.
- It can detect some abnormalities.
- The position of the baby and the placenta. If they find that the placenta is low, later in pregnancy, it may mean you are advised to have a caesarian section.
- To make sure that the baby is growing as expected. This is important for all pregnancies, but considered more so if you're carrying twins or you have experienced problems in this or a previous pregnancy.

The first ultrasound is carried out at 8 to 14 weeks, and is used to confirm your due date, based on your baby's measurements. The scan usually lasts about 20 minutes, but don't worry if the sonographer can't get a good view. It is normally because the baby is moving around, or is in an awkward position. Also, the ultrasound quality may not be as clear, if you are overweight or your body tissue is dense. It may take longer for the ultrasound, or you may need to have a repeat scan. The sonographer may also do what is known as a 'nuchal translucency test'. This is part of the screening test for Down Syndrome.

The second ultrasound is carried out at 18 to 21 weeks, and is used to detect abnormalities or irregularities. Some women may have more than two scans, and this is usually due to either an issue with their health, or the health of their baby. Someone can accompany you to the scan, although you may not want to take young children with you. If you want to know the sex of the baby, you can usually do so at the 18 to 21-week scan.

NB: It is not always possible for the sonographer to confirm the baby's sex, and some hospitals may have a policy of not telling you. Ask your midwife or sonographer for more information.

What blood tests will you have?
Blood tests are a routine part of antenatal care, and they give you and your midwife or doctor important information on your health, and that of your baby. At your first booking appointment, you will be offered some, or all these tests. If you don't understand what a certain test is for, ask your midwife or doctor to explain. As with a scan, only you can decide if you want to have the blood tests:

a) Blood Group:
This is in case you require a blood transfusion during pregnancy, or labour.

b) Haemoglobin:
This detects whether the level of haemoglobin in your blood is low, which means you have iron deficiency anaemia. Your body needs iron to produce haemoglobin, which in turn carries oxygen around your body in red blood cells.

If you are anaemic, your midwife/doctor will advise what foods eat to boost your iron levels. They may also prescribe iron tablets.

c) Rhesus Factor:
If a person's blood shows that they are rhesus positive, it means they have a certain protein on the surface of their red blood cells. If you are rhesus negative but the baby's father is rhesus positive, there is a chance the baby will be positive too. If this is the case, your body may start to produce antibodies that attack the baby's red blood cells. You can be given an injection of an antibody called immunoglobulin, at 28 weeks. Ask your midwife/doctor for more details

d) Hepatitis B:
If you pass hepatitis B on to your baby, before or after they are born, they need to be started on a series of injections (vaccine and antibodies) as soon as they are born. Your doctor will carry out a blood test, when your child reaches one, to see if they have avoided infection.

e) Syphilis:
Thankfully this sexually transmitted disease is rare nowadays. But if you do have it and it isn't treated, while you are pregnant, it could cause abnormalities in your baby. Syphilis can also cause a baby to be stillborn. The blood test can sometimes produce a false-positive result. This is because the syphilis bacteria and other bacteria (that cause non-sexually transmitted diseases) can look similar. If you do have syphilis, you will be treated with penicillin. This might be

enough to prevent your baby from contracting the disease but some may need antibiotics after birth.

f) HIV/AIDS:
All mums-to-be are offered a blood test to detect HIV/AIDS. You can turn it down if you want to. However, if the doctors know you have the virus, steps can be taken to reduce the chance of the virus being transmitted to your baby.

g) Blood Tests for Other Disorders
In most cases, sickle-cell disorders are more likely in people of African and African-Caribbean descent, while Thalassaemia is more common in people of Asian or Mediterranean origin. If you come from these backgrounds you should be offered a test for sickle-cell or thalassaemia at your booking appointment. They can make you anaemic, and can be passed on to your baby. In most parts of the UK, all pregnant women are offered a test for thalassaemia. But there are different approaches to screening for sickle-cell disease, depending on how prevalent the condition is in the area. All pregnant women should be offered screening, in areas where there is a high number of cases.

Furthermore, all pregnant women should be offered a screening test for genetic abnormalities e.g. Down syndrome. One of the most accurate tests is the combined screening test. This consists of blood tests and the nuchal translucency scan, mentioned earlier, that is done at your dating scan. This is now recommended throughout the UK, as it gives a more reliable risk rating (whether your baby may have problems).

Screening tests can't tell you 100% that your baby has a problem. If you want to be certain, you need to go on to have diagnostic tests such as chorionic villus sampling or amniocentesis. These will be discussed with you if it is found on the combined screening test that your baby may have problems.

Not all women need all blood tests. Many factors come into play when deciding what and when to test. You need to discuss with your midwife/doctor which tests are right for you.

Chapter 5

Nutrition in Pregnancy

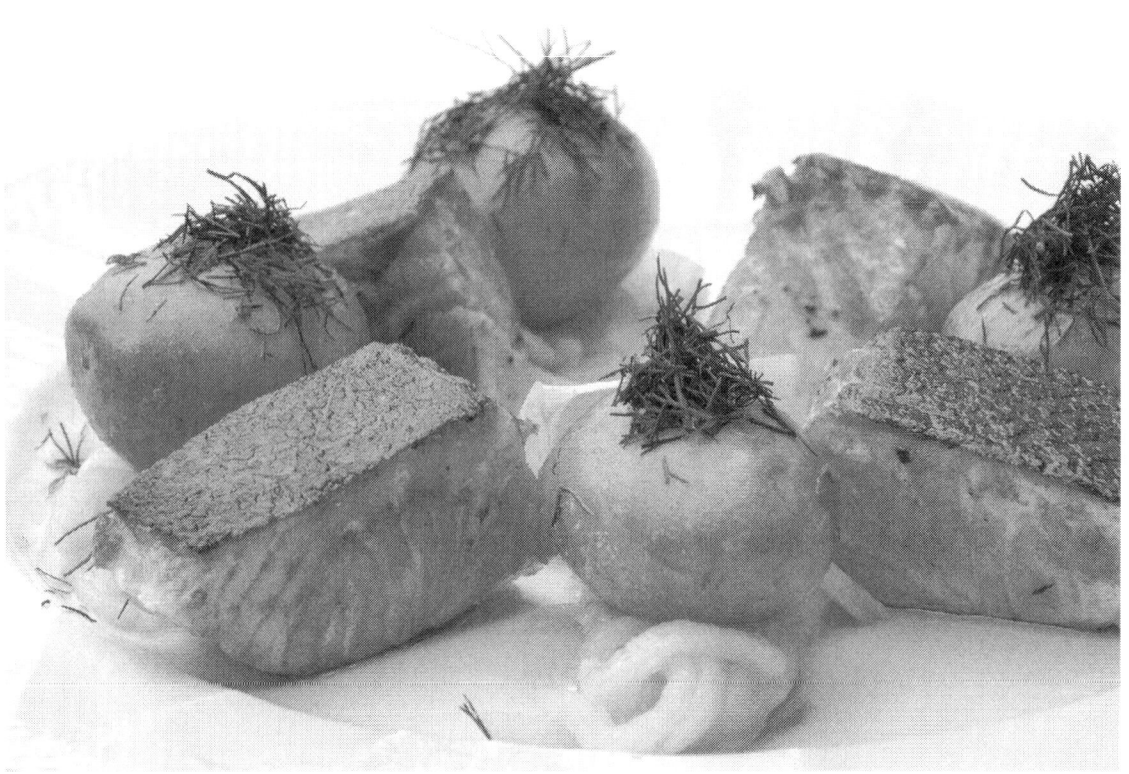

A healthy diet should be a part of daily life, whether pregnant or not. Nutrition plays an important role in pregnancy, and you need to remember the foetus is connected to you by the placenta and receives all its nutrients via the umbilical cord.

If you have any specific dietary concerns based on factors such as religious/ethical beliefs; medical issues (e.g. allergies), please make an appointment to see your health professional prior to, or as soon after conception as possible. They can then help you plan a healthy diet, tailored to your specific needs or refer you to a dietician if necessary.

Above all, you need to follow a healthy diet and your body needs extra vitamins and minerals but there is no need to 'eat for two'. It is advised that you eat an extra 350 to 500 calories (1470 to 2090 kilo-joules) during the 2nd and 3rd trimesters only. If your diet is lacking, it may affect the baby's development, also poor eating habits and excess weight gain puts you at higher risk of gestational diabetes, or birth complications.

It is important that your baby gets a good supply of nutrients. The following should make up the basis of your healthy diet.

a) Fruits and vegetables:
There are vitamins, minerals and fibre in fruits and vegetables, that ensure healthy growth in your baby, and aid digestion and prevent constipation in you. It is advised you eat at least 5 portions of fruit and vegetables a day. Leafy green vegetables such as broccoli and kale contain folate and vitamin B6. You should have been taking folic acid prior to pregnancy and up until week 12, and you may be taking antenatal vitamins that contain folic acid (folate).

However, eating foods containing folate is a plus. Other fruit and veg that contain folate and vitamin B are: Citrus fruits, dried beans, peas. Make sure you always wash fruit and vegetables carefully. If abroad wash them using bottled or cooled, boiled water, as the tap water may be contaminated.

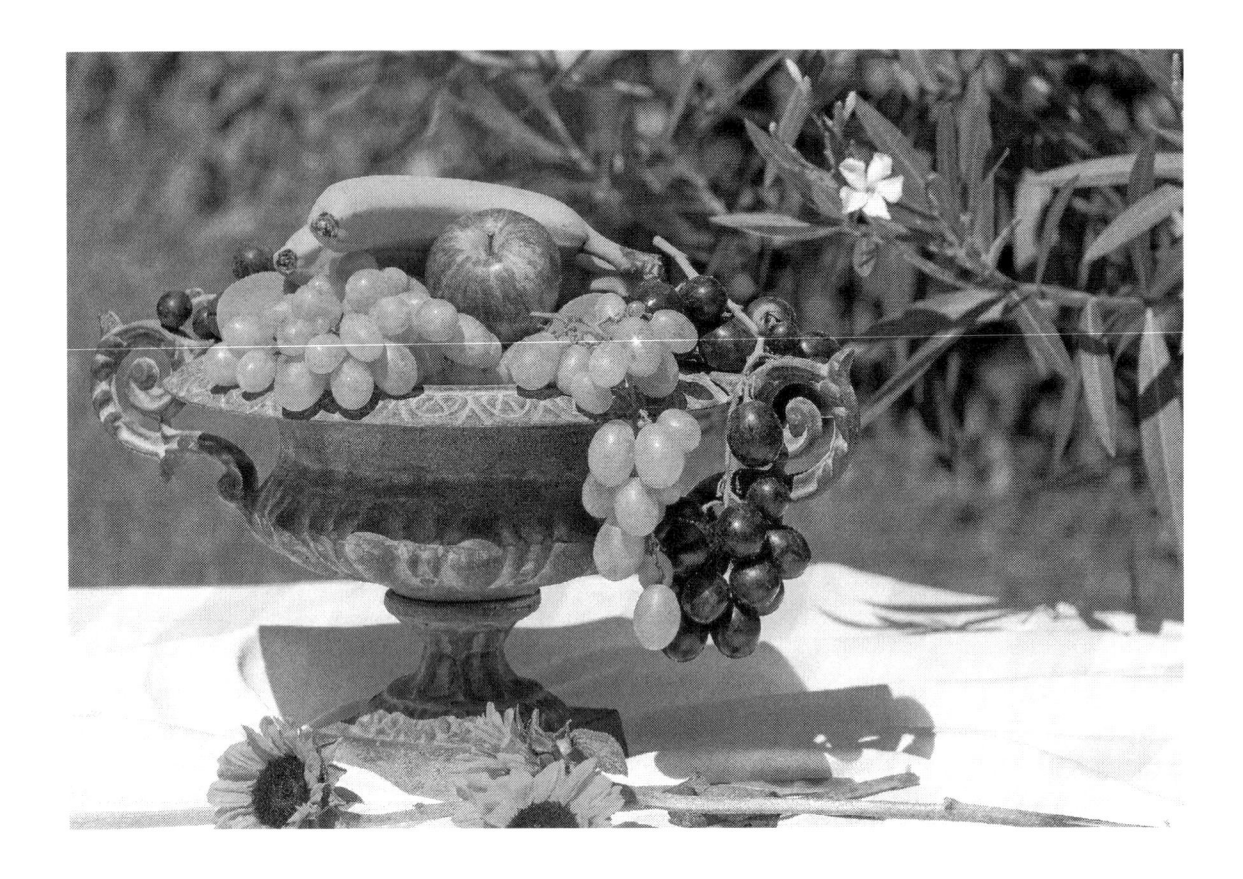

b) Protein:

Needs to be a part of your daily diet. Sources of protein include fish, meat (avoid liver), poultry, eggs, beans, pulses and nuts. Choose lean meat and remove the skin for poultry when cooking, and try to use little or no oil when cooking. You need to make sure that all meat, fish, eggs etc. are cooked thoroughly. If you can, eat at least 2 portions of fish a week (one should be an oily fish like mackerel). Please see the section below for meat to avoid.

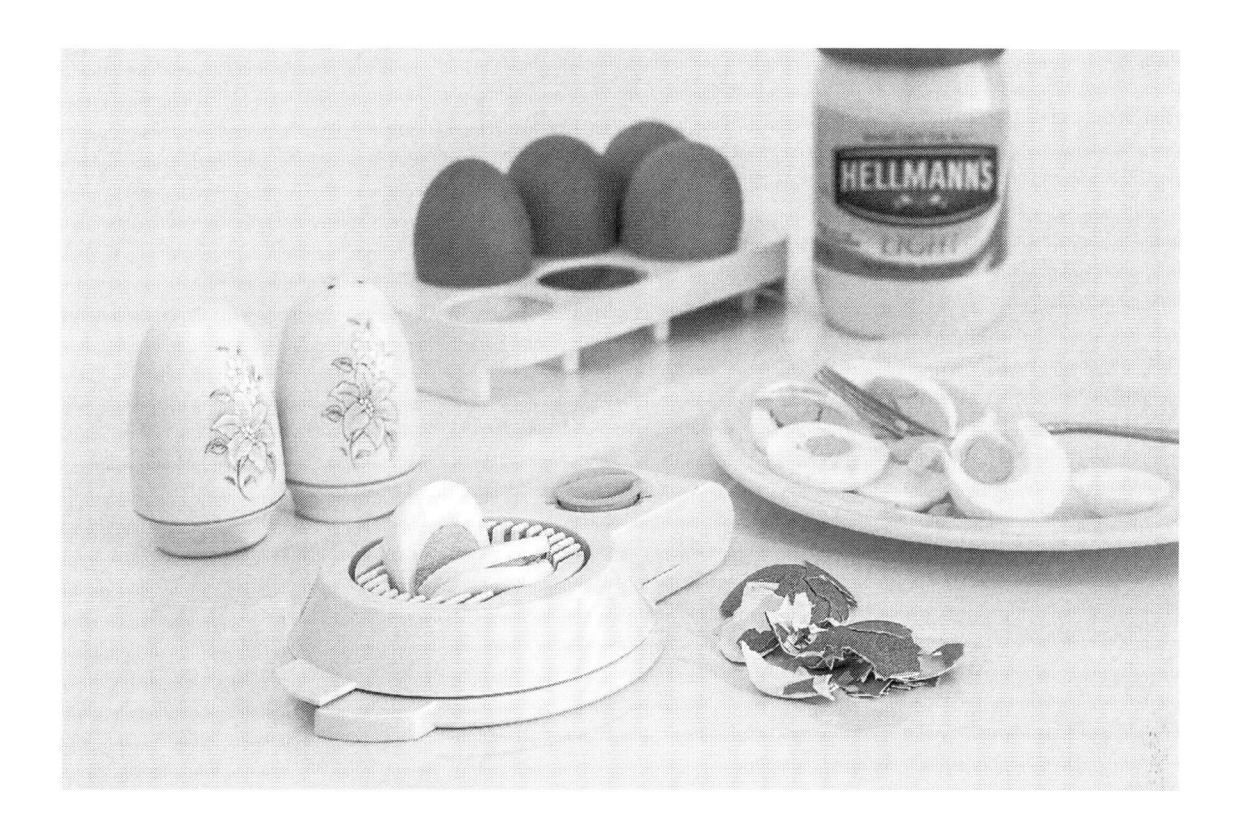

c) **Carbohydrates (starchy foods):**

These are important for energy, certain vitamins and fibre. They should make up a third of your diet and can help fill you up, and if you choose wisely should not contain too many calories. These include bread, potatoes, breakfast cereal, pasta, oats and rice. Swap refined, white options for wholegrain, high fibre options.

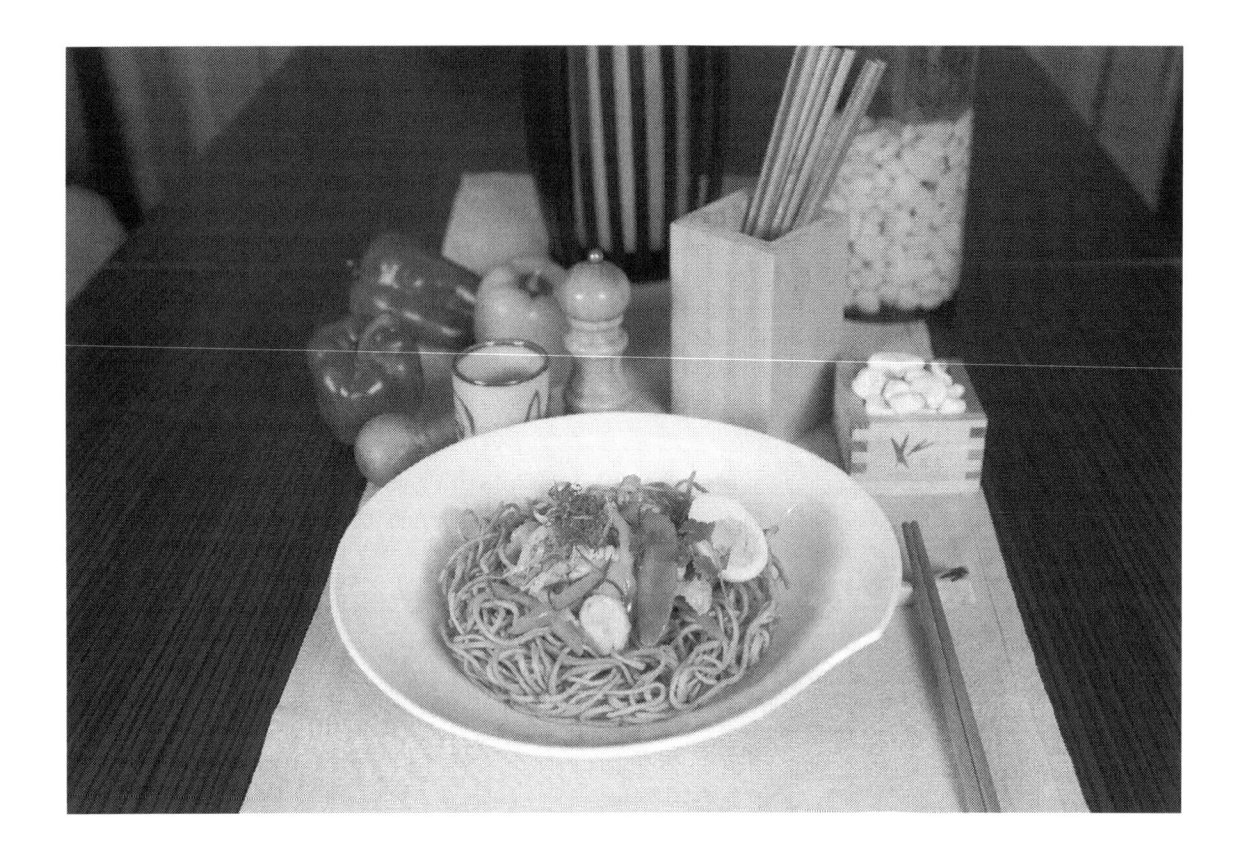

d) Dairy Foods:

Milk, cheese, yoghurt etc. are important in pregnancy as they provide you and baby with calcium. Try to choose lower fat options (you still receive the required amount of calcium). If you do not eat dairy you can substitute with soya drinks etc. Please see the section below for cheeses to avoid in pregnancy.

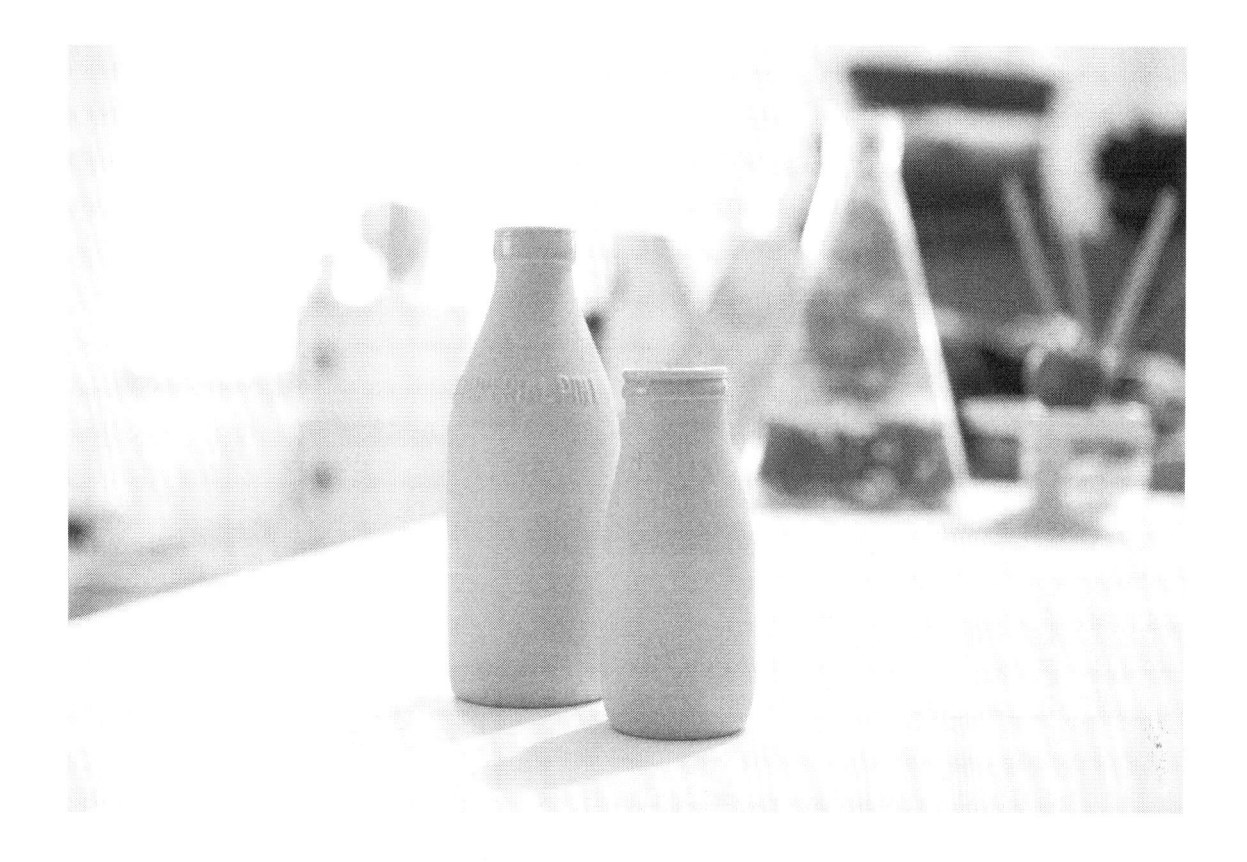

e) Iron:

Legumes such as, lentils, kidney beans, black beans and chick peas, are a great source of iron. You and your baby use a lot iron during pregnancy, and it is important to keep replenishing the supply. It is better to consume iron in food, than to take iron supplements, as these can lead to constipation.

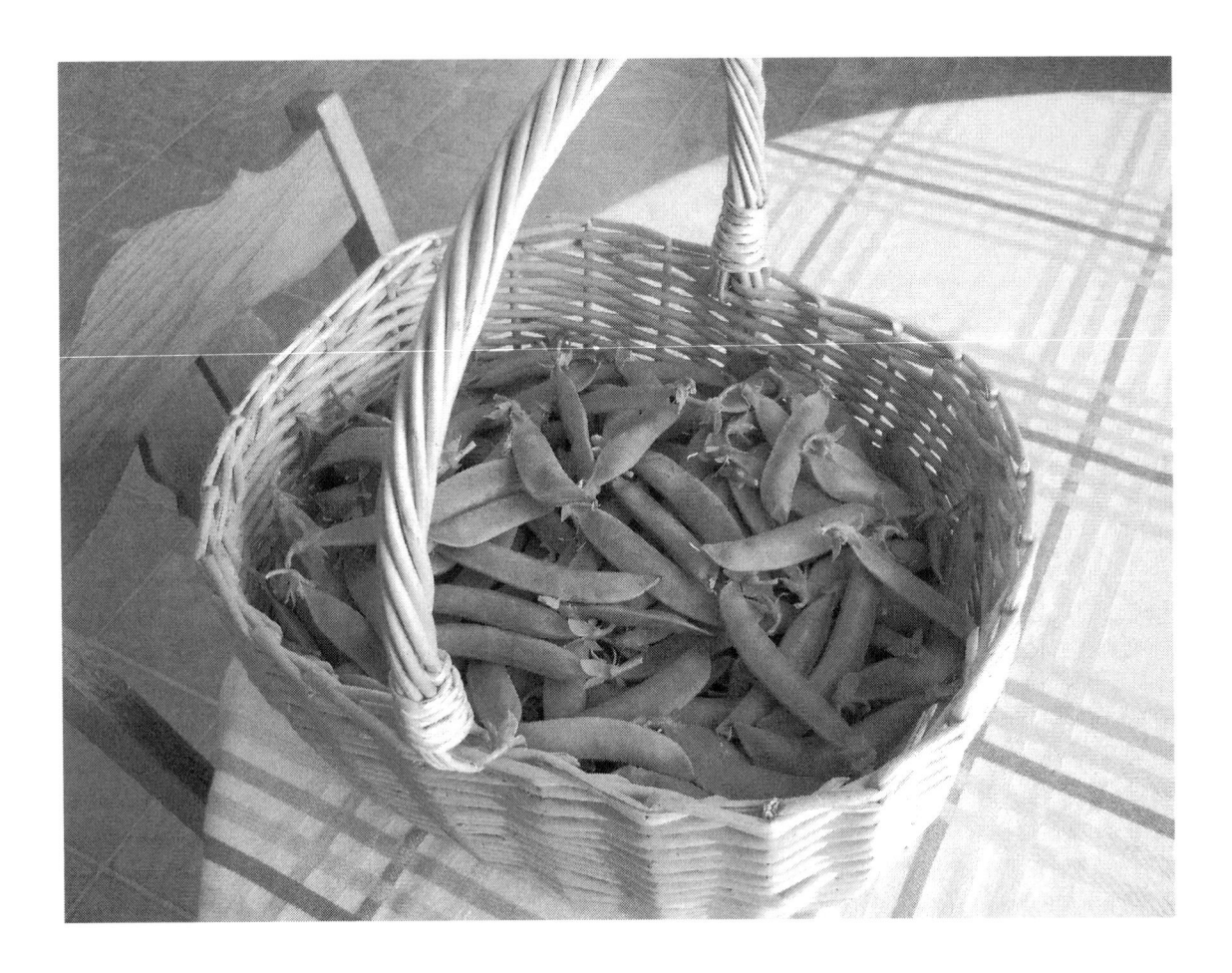

Some foods (high in fat and sugar) should be consumed in moderation throughout your pregnancy, as they can lead to excess weight gain. This is not good for either you or your baby, as it can lead to pregnancy complications, like gestational diabetes. These include but are not limited to: Oils; spreads (margarine or butter); chocolate; crisps; cake; biscuits; deserts. No-one is saying they should be completely banned but they should be consumed less often and in small amounts!

What foods should I avoid during pregnancy?

It is recommended you do not eat the following:

a) Certain cheese:

Soft pasteurised cheeses e.g. camembert, mozzarella. These can contain listeria (a bacteria) that can harm your unborn baby. Stick to eating hard cheese varieties, like cheddar or edam.

b) Cream and custard:

You should avoid pre-prepared foods e.g. bakery items with custard or cream used as an ingredient. Also, avoid ready-made supermarket custard.

c) Hummus:

It is best to avoid store bought hummus and other pre-packaged, chilled dips. They may contain bacteria that are harmful to your baby. Homemade hummus/dips are generally considered safe. Just ensure you store them in the fridge (in an air-tight container) and use within a couple of days.

d) Pate:

This too can contain listeria (vegetable pâté isn't safe either.)

e) Raw or partially cooked eggs:

Eggs can contain salmonella, which is a major cause of food poisoning. When pregnant, avoid any food that contains uncooked egg e.g. homemade mayonnaise. You don't need to avoid eggs completely, as they're a great source of protein. Just make sure that both the yolk and white are well cooked.

f) Raw, cured and undercooked meat:

Raw, undercooked, or cured meats like ham and pepperoni, increase the risk of food poisoning and parasitic infections, and can affect your baby's development. You also need to be extra careful how you cook chicken, as it can contain salmonella and other bacteria. It should be well cooked, all the way through. Be careful of smoked salmon, as it hasn't been through traditional cooking processes and can carry bacteria. It's a good idea to avoid this during pregnancy.

g) Liver:

Liver contains high levels of Vitamin A, which in large quantities can harm your baby. You need to be careful with vitamin or mineral supplements during pregnancy. If you think you need supplements, discuss this with your GP.

h) Some types of fish:

Fish is a fantastic source of vitamins, minerals and protein, and is also high in omega 3 fatty acids, which help your baby's nervous system develop. Most common types of fish are safe. However, some contain higher levels of Mercury and other pollutants. If you have any doubts about whether a type of fish is safe to eat please talk to your midwife/doctor or see a dietician.

i) Raw shellfish:

Reduce the risk of food poisoning by not eating raw shellfish and making sure any shellfish you do eat is thoroughly cooked.

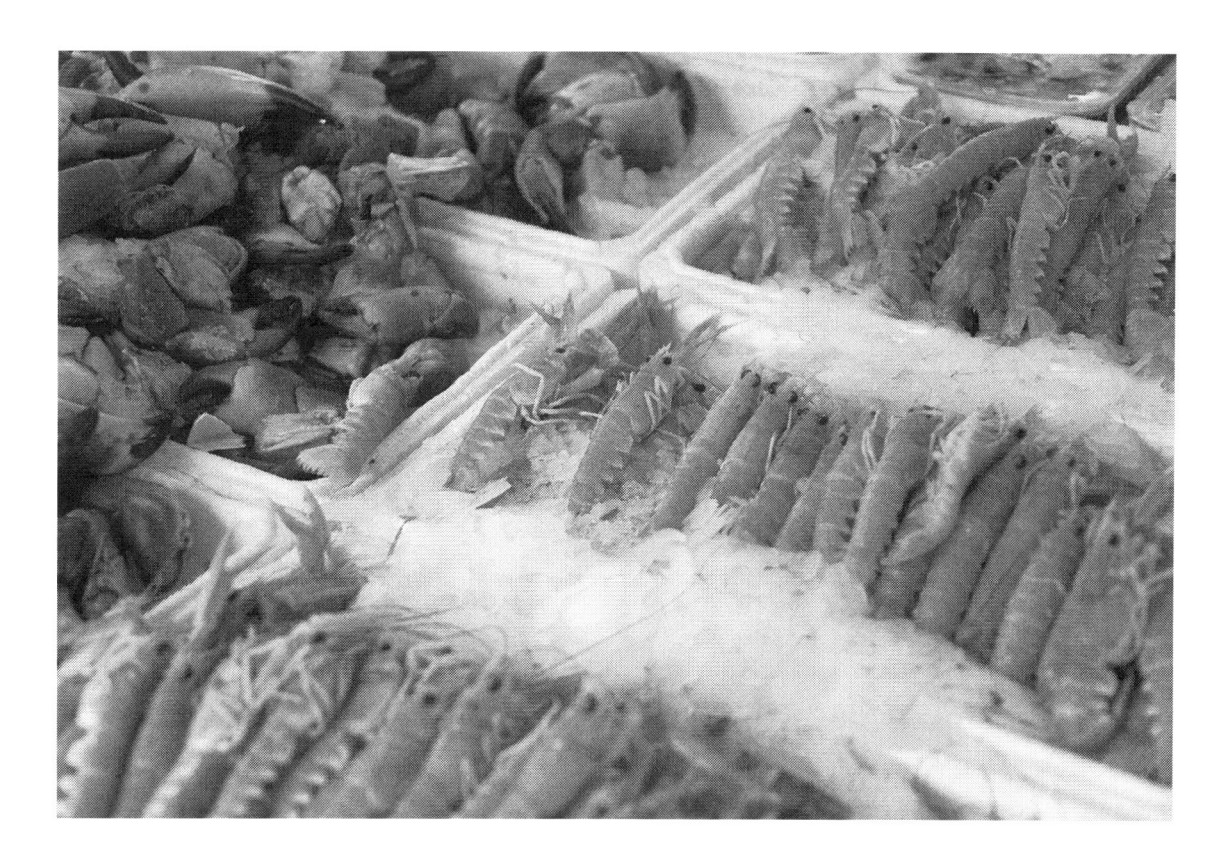

j) Pre-prepared chilled meals and leftovers:

Keep all cooked foods in the fridge and ensure you cook them at high temperatures to kill bacteria. The food should be piping hot right the way through.

k) Caffeine:

Drinking an excess of caffeine can lead to low birth weight, and it has also been linked to miscarriages. It is best to limit your intake of caffeine or alternatively choose decaffeinated versions of your favourite hot drinks. Pregnant and breastfeeding women are advised to limit their caffeine intake to a maximum of 300mg per day. This is roughly equivalent to 4 cups of plunger coffee, 6 cups of instant coffee, or 6 cups of tea, or 400g plain chocolate!

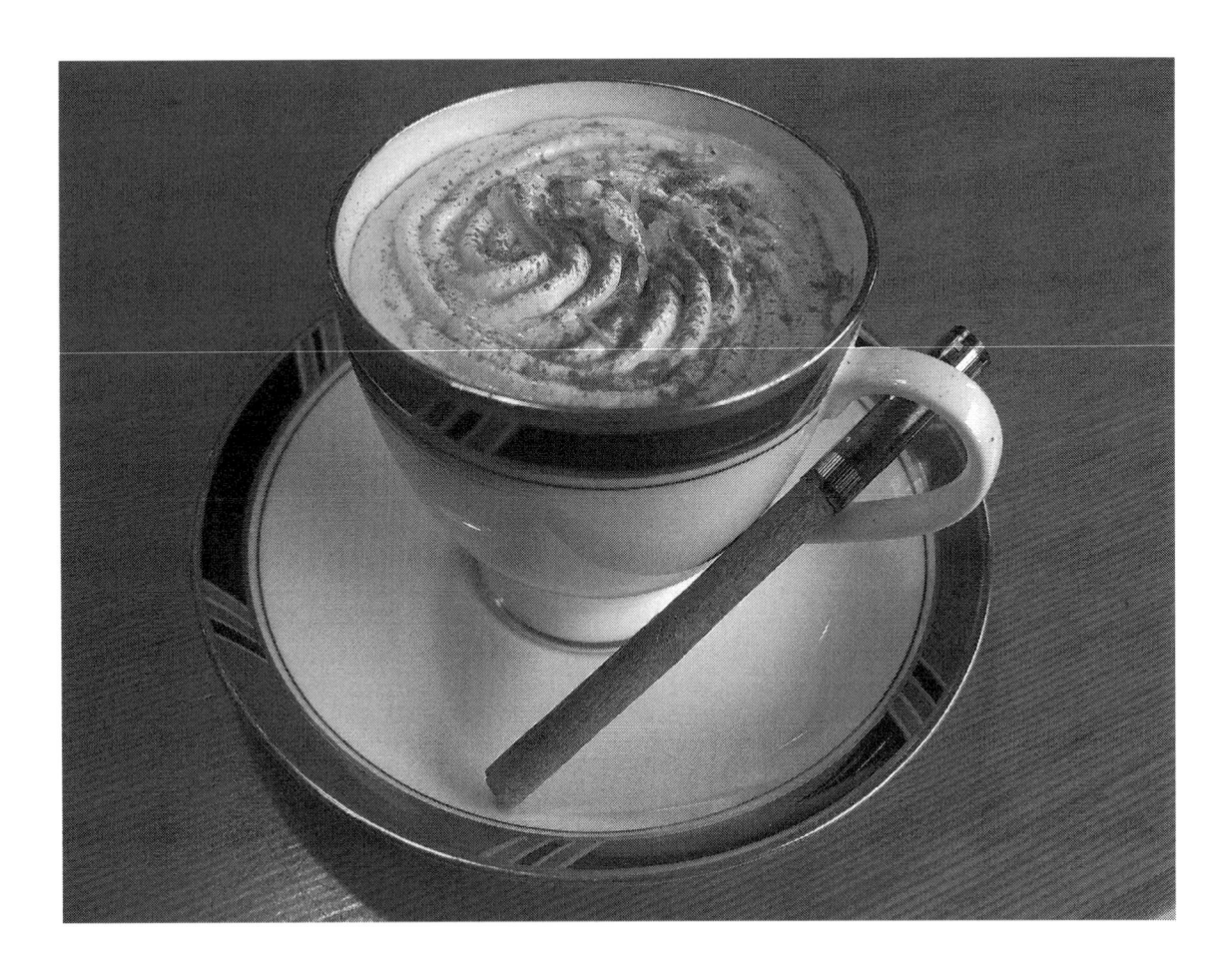

1) Sushi:

It is best to avoid sushi made with raw fish, while trying to conceive or pregnant.

Raw fish can contain bacteria and viruses that are harmful to you and your baby.

Stick to sushi made with cooked meat or vegetables.

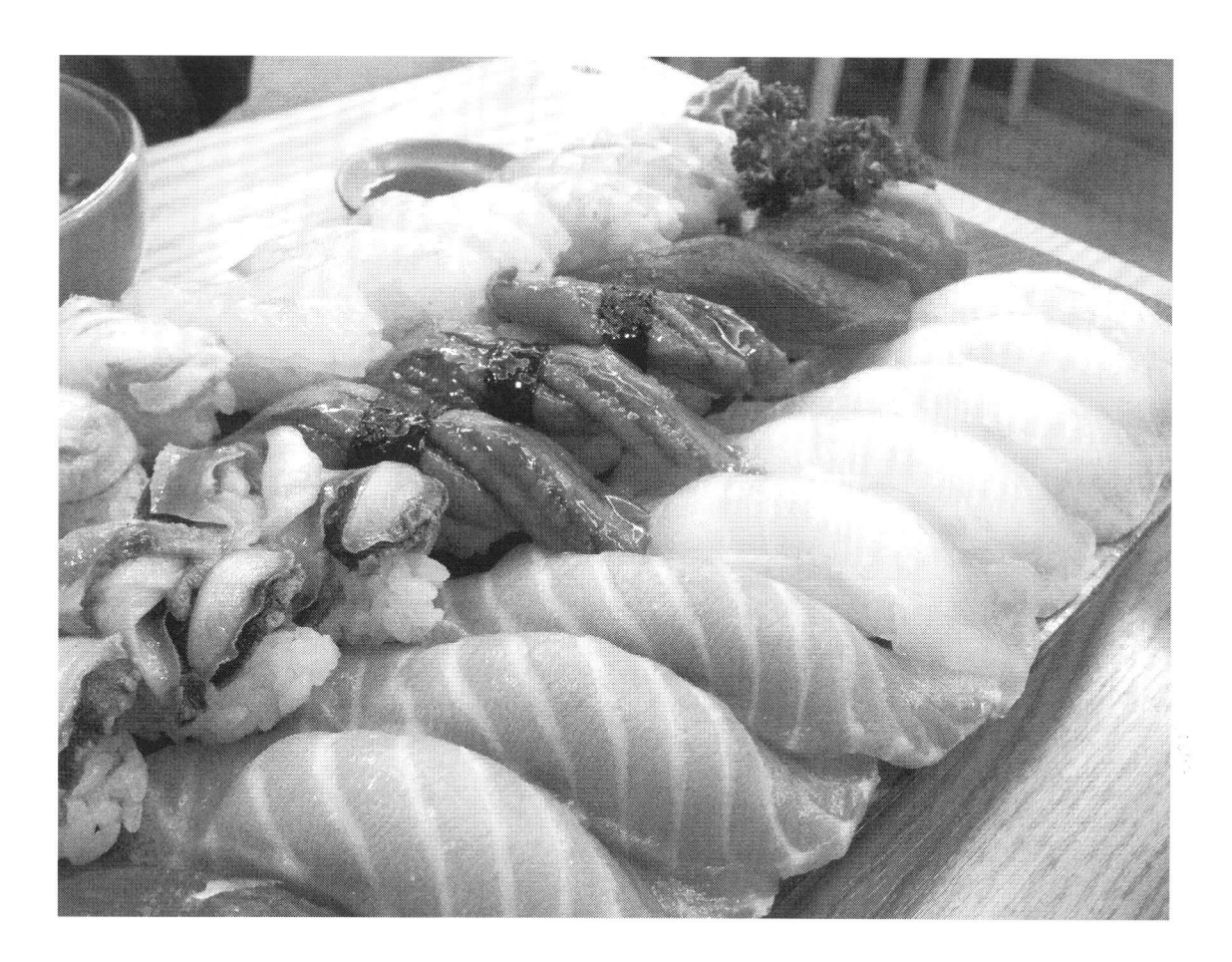

Chapter 6

Weight Gain and Exercise During Pregnancy

Pregnancy can make the fittest of us conscious of our size, especially if they are having a multiple pregnancy. Not every body type is the same and weight gain differs from woman to woman. Before pregnancy a woman fits into a specific category with regards to their weight. It depends on a woman's pre-pregnancy weight and Body Mass Index (BMI), how much weight should be gained during pregnancy. Below shows a woman's pre-pregnancy BMI, and their estimated weight gain.

Pre-pregnancy BMI	BMI	Total weight gain
Underweight	Less than 18.5	13kg to 18kg (28lb to 40lb)
Normal weight	18.5 to 24.9	11.5kg to 16kg (25lb to 35lb)
Overweight	25 to 29.9	7kg to 11.5kg (15lb to 25lb)
Obese	30 or more	5kg to 9kg (11lb to 20lb)

NB: This is for women who are experiencing a single pregnancy.

You will read different advice, telling you the average weight gained, in each stage of pregnancy. Some women may put on the most weight during the first 20 weeks. while others will only gain a few kilograms up until 16 weeks, then put on most in the middle of their pregnancy. All women are different and a woman's overall weight gain (carrying a single baby) can be as little as 8kg, or as much as 20kg, with an average of 12 to 14kg. Pregnancy weight gains is broken down into these factors:

Baby: 3 to 4kg

Uterus: 1kg

Amniotic fluid: 1kg

Placenta: 0.5kg

Increase in blood volume: 1.5kg

Breasts: 0.5kg

Fat stored in preparation for breast feeding: 3.5kg

Fluid retention: 1.5kg

Once your baby is born, breastfeeding can help you lose some of the baby weight, but keep in mind that it can normally take up to a year to lose all the baby weight.

Exercise is an important part of life, and just as an important part of a healthy pregnancy. In moderation and with some exceptions, exercise you did before becoming pregnant can continue to be enjoyed throughout pregnancy. So, if you were not a marathon runner before becoming pregnant, now is probably not the time to start! Always talk to your midwife or doctor about exercising, whilst pregnant. When exercising, it is important to keep hydrated and be sensible.

Skipping meals is never a good idea when pregnant. Your baby needs extra nutrients, so it is better to skip a workout than a meal.

There are a variety of exercises, appropriate to participate in whilst pregnant. So, if you enjoy swimming, walking, yoga, and Pilates, you will benefit from continuing these in pregnancy. As your pregnancy progresses your body may tell you to slow down, a hint you may need to stop the Zumba classes!

Not all exercise is advised during pregnancy. Although there may not be direct evidence to advise against a particular form of pregnancy, it is often due to the fact that the particular exercise puts you more at risk or falls or other injury. These can include, but are not limited to, the following:

Bikram yoga (Hot yoga):
This is done in a heated environment. There hasn't been any specific research done to find out its effects. It is advised that you avoid doing exercise that raises your core body temperature more than 2 degreesC, This is reduce the chance of neural tube defects e.g. spina bifida

Horse riding, gymnastics and cycling:
As pregnancy progresses your centre of gravity changes due to your baby bump. You are at an increased risk of falling, so you are advised to avoid these forms of exercise, and any other activities that may put you at risk (e.g. climbing ladders).

Contact sports:
For example, football, martial arts, hockey. These put you at risk because you may receive a direct blow to your bump, which may cause injury to the baby.

Scuba diving:
This needs to be avoided during pregnancy, as your baby is not protected against getting decompression sickness ('the bends') or a gas embolus (bubble in the blood, that may cut off the blood supply, or cause difficulty breathing). Scuba diving has been linked to birth defects.

Other do's and don'ts

- Don't position your 'baby bump' in any awkward positions.
- You will probably want to avoid lying flat after 16 week. Your 'bump' will press on blood vessels, reducing cardiac (heart) output. You may feel dizzy and the blood flow to the baby is affected. Try laying on your side.
- You should not participate in any activity where you hold your breath.
- Do not exercise in heat or humid conditions

NB: If you experience any bleeding or cramping while exercising stop immediately, and contact your health professional.

Postnatally

The first six weeks after delivery should be reserved for healing. You may be feeling very tired, so don't do too much, too soon. Try to wait until after your postnatal check, at between six and eight weeks after the birth, before taking up any exercise other than walking.

A Caesarian section is a major operation! You should not push yourself too soon. Again, the first six weeks are needed for healing, and you should not do any strenuous exercise in the first couple of months. Even heavy lifting at home should be avoided.

Chapter 7

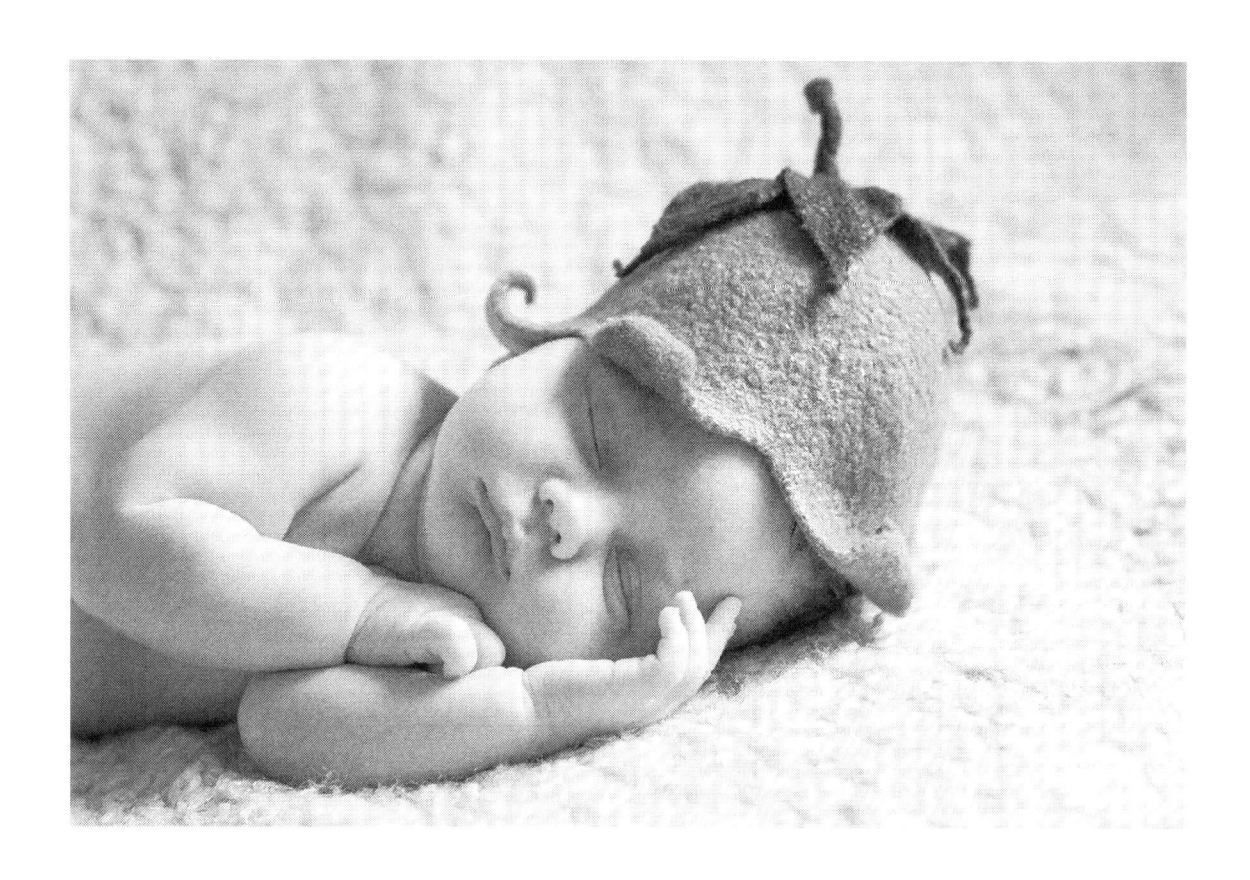

Embryo and Foetal Development

You and your baby's development will be ongoing for the next nine months but we can break it down a little. Remember your weeks of pregnancy are dated from the first date of your last period, so for the first week or so you are not actually pregnant.

Week 3:
You will release an egg about 2 weeks after your last period. During week 3 the fertilized egg moves along the fallopian tube towards your womb (uterus). It

starts off as a single cell but divides over and over. When it reaches your uterus, it is a about 100 cells called an embryo, and implants in the womb lining.

Weeks 4 to 5:
This is usually when women suspect they may be pregnant. The embryo is now two layers of cells and about 2mm long. In the outer layer is a hollow tube that has a groove/folds that develops into the brain and spinal cord. The nervous system is starting to develop, as are the foundations that will be the baby's heart and circulatory system. They also have some of their own blood vessels, and are connected to you by some that will go on to become the umbilical cord.

Week 6:
There is a bulge where the heart is and a bump at one end. This bump becomes the brain and head. Your baby's face will begin to take shape, there are dimples where the ears will be, and a slight thickening in the place where their eyes are.

Week 8:
The embryo is now called a 'foetus' (which means offspring in Latin), weighs 1 gram and is 1.6 cm in length and starts to move around inside your uterus. The nerve cells continue to multiply, and the nervous system begins to form. The inner ear starts to develop but it takes another few weeks for the outer ear to do so. The buds where arms and legs will be, grow longer, and start to form cartilage.

Week 10:
By now your baby's face is starting to form, as the eyes are bigger and more noticeable. The mouth has developed with a tongue that has tiny taste buds, and ears start to develop at the side of the head. Hands and feet are developing and there are fingers and toes, but these are webbed in appearance. All the major organs continue to develop, and the heart is fully formed and beats about 180 times a minute.

Week 12:
Your baby is around 5.4 cm and weighs 14 grams. All their limbs, bones, organs, muscles and sex organs are in place. Their eyelids remain closed and won't open for a few more months. Up until now the bones have been formed of cartilage but now bone begins to develop. From now on, they need to mature and grow.

Weeks 13 to 16:
By the end of week 16 your baby will weigh about 140g and be 13cm approximately. The sex organs on the inside are fully developed and the genitals now start to form externally. They start to swallow amniotic fluid, and their kidneys begin to work, so fluid will pass back into the fluid as urine. Their eyes begin to be sensitive to light, and although they remain closed they can register if there is bright light. The nervous system has continued to develop, along with muscle control. They can now reach with their hands and even grasp them together.

Weeks 17 to 20:
By the end of 20 weeks they weigh about 300g and are approximately 27cm long. Their facial features take on a more human appearance and they have eyelids and eyebrows. They can move their eyes but their eyelids remain closed. Fingerprints are now present, making them a unique person, and finger and toe nails are growing. Baby is now moving around a lot, and this is when you may start to feel them. A lot of women say it feels like 'butterflies in their tummy', its official term is 'quickening'. They will respond to loud music or bangs. They continue to put on weight throughout but at this stage they don't have much of a fat store, so appear a little wrinkled. 'Vernix' appears at around 20 weeks, which is a waxy like substance, that can help to protect newborns from infection. It contains antioxidants, anti-inflammatory and antibacterial properties.

Weeks 21 to 24:
At the end of 24 weeks, your baby will weigh approximately 660 grams and be 34.6cm long. From now onwards they will weigh more than the placenta. They develop a more defined waking and sleep pattern, and unfortunately this is not always the same as you! Their lungs are not yet full formed but they start to practice breathing for when they are born. They are covered in a soft, very fine hair which is called 'lanugo'. It is not 100% known why it is present but may have something to do with temperature regulation, and it usually disappears before birth.

Week 25 to 28:
Your baby will weigh 1.15kg at the end of 27 weeks, and they continue to put on weight, due to fat now appearing under their skin. Their systems are fully formed but need time to mature. Your midwife/doctor will be able to hear their heartbeat through a stethoscope, and it will beat at about 100 beats each minute. They will now move rapidly and may respond to your touch. Their eyelids open around this time and they start blinking. They continue to swallow the amniotic fluid, produce urine and may start to get hiccoughs (hiccups), which you may feel!

Weeks 29 to 32:
By the end of 32 weeks they will be approximately 1.92kg and 44cm in length. Your baby continues to be very active, and you will become aware of their patterns in movement. Every baby has their own pattern, so don't worry if yours differs to another pregnant woman. The vernix and lanugo start to decrease in amount. Their sucking reflex has now started to develop, so they can suck their fingers or thumb, and their eyes can focus. The lungs continue to develop but they are not usually able to breathe unaided until they reach 36 week's gestation. By this time, you may find your baby turns to face downward, in readiness for birth. This is known as a 'cephalic presentation'. Don't be concerned if they haven't, as there is still time.

NB: If you notice any change in your baby's movement pattern or you have any concerns, contact your GP/Midwife.

Weeks 33 to 36:
By the end of week 36 your baby will be considered full term and weighs around 3 to 4 kg. By this stage the following are fully formed and the baby is ready to take their first breath: brain and nervous system; bones (apart from skull); if it's a boy the testicles begin to descend into the scrotum; digestive system is prepared to cope with breast milk. There is little room for your baby to move, but they will still change position. You may even be able to see them move through your skin!

NB: The skull bones remain soft and separate until after birth so it makes it easier for the baby to travel through the birth canal. They slide over each other, while still protecting the brain.

Weeks 37 to 40:
In a few weeks, it will be time to meet your baby, exciting! If it hasn't happened before, then the baby should turn to face downwards and move down into your pelvis, this is called 'engaged'. You may notice your bump move down a little bit. The lanugo should almost have disappeared. The hormones in your system may cause your baby's genitalia to appear swollen when they are born. This will soon settle down. Your baby's digestive system will now contain a substance called 'meconium'. It is sticky and green, and will be your baby's first poo. If your baby does a poo, while you are in labour, the amniotic fluid will have meconium in it. The midwife will want to keep a closer eye on you, as it can mean the baby is in distress.

N.B: If you experience any of the following signs during late pregnancy, make sure you contact your health professional immediately:

- Vaginal bleeding (could signal a serious problem e.g. placental abruption)
- High blood pressure or protein in your urine (pre-eclampsia)
- Itching (at any stage of pregnancy) could indicate a rare pregnancy complication called 'Obstetric Cholestasis'. It is caused by a build-up of bile acids in the blood stream, which causes the itch, and may result in pregnancy complications.

Chapter 8

Changes During Pregnancy

What happens to your body while pregnant? It is obvious that your body is going through changes but emotions also tend to undergo change, due to the influence of hormones. But how exactly does your body change to accommodate the baby?

Respiratory System
Your respiratory (breathing) system sends oxygenated blood throughout your body to keep vital organs healthy and working correctly. While you are pregnant, you may notice changes to your respiratory system, to compensate for the oxygen demands of your uterus, foetus, and placenta. You may have a feeling of being breathless, from walking or going up-and-down stairs.

Cardiovascular System
During pregnancy, your body needs to adjust to an increased demand on your cardiovascular (heart) system, to meet the demands of both mother and foetus. There is a blood volume increase, of about 40 to 50%, to ensure your baby is receiving sufficient oxygen and nutrients. In addition to the increased blood volume, there is also an increase in maternal heartrate of 15 beats per minute.

Gastrointestinal System
Your uterus increases in size to accommodate an ever-growing baby. It rises from where it usually sits, in the pelvic cavity, and when this happens, your intestines, stomach, and other organs are displaced. The hormone, progesterone causes

your lower oesophageal sphincter to relax. This means you may experience: heartburn, constipation and acid reflux.

Endocrine System

Hormonal changes may cause the following:

- Your parathyroid gland increases production of calcium to keep up with you and your baby's demands.

- You may experience hot flushes, thanks to the increase of hormone levels. There is also a significant increase in your basal metabolic rate (the amount of energy the body uses at rest).

- While you are pregnant, the baby's placenta acts as a temporary endocrine gland. This helps produce the large amounts of oestrogen and progesterone your body requires by weeks 10 and 12 of pregnancy. It is also helps to maintain the growth of your uterus and controls uterine activity.

Uterus

Your uterus gradually expands throughout pregnancy. Before pregnancy it is a pear-shaped organ and approximately 4.5cm x 7.6cm and 3cm thick; by 20-22 weeks it reaches the umbilicus (belly button); at full-term it is the size of a watermelon! As you approach your second trimester, you will begin to see changes in your abdomen as your baby grows and your uterus expands to allow the room. It is possible that you may begin to feel an ache, on one side of your abdominal wall, where your ligaments are stretching to support your uterus.

Urinary System

You've probably heard that pregnant women 'wee' what seems like every five minutes! As explained previously, in early pregnancy this is caused by hormonal changes. Later as your uterus expands and exerts pressure on your bladder, pelvic floor muscles, and urethra. You may even experience some leakage of urine when you laugh, cough or sneeze. This is normal and not something to worry about, but be sure to practice your pelvic floor exercises.

Musculoskeletal System

Your bones also change in pregnancy. There is realignment to the curve in your spine, to allow you to keep your balance as your tummy gets bigger. You will feel a shift in posture, that leads to the 'typical gait' you see in women in the late stages of pregnancy. Ligaments become relaxed, due to a hormone called 'relaxin', and this contributes to the back and pubic pain you feel closer to your due date.

Skin

Some women have a certain 'glow' when they get to a point in pregnancy. You may notice hyperpigmentation in a line down the centre of your abdomen (linea nigra), nipples, and even your face. This is caused by hormonal changes that are occurring in your body.

Spider veins

These are small, visible red blood vessels, and do look a little like spiders. They are due to an increase in blood circulating through your body, plus hormonal changes.

Varicose vein

You may get varicose veins during pregnancy, due to an increase in blood volume and your uterus putting pressure on the large vein (inferior vena cava), on the right side of your body. This in turn puts extra pressure on the veins in your legs. Some tips that may help to prevent them are, move regularly, elevate your legs when resting, watch your weight and sleep on your left side.

Stretch marks

These can be common in pregnant women and will most likely occur during the second half of your pregnancy. You will begin to see them on your thighs, abdomen, breasts and even buttocks. Stretch marks are just scars that occur when the skin is stretched beyond what is normal, thanks to the growing baby.

Breasts

Breasts change to allow you to breast feed your baby when they are born (if you so choose). Until your milk comes in after giving birth, you will experience some of these changes, as you progress through pregnancy. Your breasts will become larger and more sensitive, due to the increased levels of oestrogen and progesterone, in your system; your nipples may be more pronounced; the areolas around your nipple will darken and enlarge; colostrum may leak from your nipples; your breasts produce colostrum – this starts in pregnancy and continues in the early days of breastfeeding. Colostrum is low in fat but high in antibodies, protein and calcium and is designed to get your baby off to a healthy start.

Other changes

You may notice an increase in your body temperature in early pregnancy. When you get to around the sixteenth week of gestation, your temperature should start to return to normal.

Cramp in your legs is common, due to fatigue carrying around the extra pregnancy weight. It causes compression in the blood vessels of your legs. This can also occur due to a shortage of calcium, magnesium or an excess of phosphorous.

Thanks to the extra fluid volume in your body, you may also begin to see swelling in your feet and ankles.

Hormones cause changes to your hair/nail texture or growth patterns. You may find your hair and nails grow faster than before you were pregnant.

Chapter 9

Pregnancy Trimesters

Your baby grows a little every day and your body is designed to keep them safe. During each stage of pregnancy, your body goes through many changes. These changes not only affect you but they have a huge impact on your baby. With each trimester comes new experiences and excitement.

Pregnancy is broken down into three trimesters or stages: First, second and third. Typically, each trimester runs for approximately three months, and the foetal stages and maternal changes will happen accordingly throughout.

First Trimester

The first trimester runs from week 0 through to the end of week 13 (month 0 to 3). Week 1 starts on the first day of your last period and you may not look pregnant but the chances are you may be feeling it. Remember the symptoms from chapter 1, these are when they may occur.

The first trimester is when you officially find out you are pregnant. However, taking care of your body before you conceive is equally important and you should already be taking folic acid. Remember you are not technically pregnant the first two weeks of your pregnancy. The first two weeks consist of your period and ovulation, and your body is preparing itself for the pregnancy process.

It is important to keep a close eye out for any unusual/unexpected symptoms that may occur during this trimester. For example, if you notice significant bleeding, severe dizziness, rapid weight gain/loss, severe abdominal pain please call your midwife/doctor, or visit a nearby hospital immediately!

Second Trimester
This starts at week 14 and runs through to week 27 (month 4 to 6)

This trimester may be the easiest of the three trimesters, as morning sickness will have hopefully have calmed, but is before your baby bump is large enough to cause discomfort.

You may begin to show; you will feel more energetic and the weight gain in this trimester is slow and steady. You may start to experience heartburn and even though you may have cravings you may not be able to indulge them.

If you have not already told family and friends you are pregnant, this may be the time to do so. Your immune system may be a little compromised, so beware of others who are unwell or have infectious illnesses. Due to the increase in the volume of blood in your body, you may experience nosebleeds, gum bleeding, or a stuffy nose.

Third Trimester
The last trimester is week 28 onwards (month 7 to 9). At the end of this trimester you will meet your new baby, however it also comes with its own special set of circumstances.

Your hands, feet, and legs may be swollen due to extra blood volume. But please be aware swelling can sometimes be a sign of preeclampsia, so if you think there is something wrong, contact your health professional immediately.

Your breasts will be larger than normal, this is due to hormonal changes and the production of colostrum. Your breasts may leak, when you least expect it, so it can be handy to have breast pads on hand.

You may experience a 'show' towards the end of pregnancy. This is the mucus plug, that seals the entrance of your uterus, slipping away. It is usually a clear, thick jelly-like substance but can be slightly tinged with blood (or old brown blood). However, if you notice any fresh bleeding with this discharge, contact your midwife/doctor.

Backache caused by your ever-expanding baby bump may be uncomfortable and annoying, and you may feel achy. Sleeping on your side, with a pillow between your knees, can help ease the backache and pains in your body.

Braxton Hicks contractions can be alarming if you don't know what they are. Some women describe Braxton Hicks contractions as a tightening in the abdomen that comes and goes, and that these "false" contractions feel like mild menstrual cramps. Braxton Hicks contractions may be uncomfortable, but they do not cause labour or open the cervix. If you are unsure about your contractions and think they may be real, call you midwife or doctor for advice.

Other symptoms during this trimester include, fatigue, heartburn, constipation, hemorrhoids, shortness of breath, spider and varicose veins, and swelling.

You are probably feeling like you are ready to explode but you are almost there. Your body is preparing for labor and if your baby has yet to turn they may do so now. At week 36, your baby's head has 'engaged' (dropped) and is preparing for its arrival into the world. You could give birth at any moment, so start to prepare things you are going to need for when the baby arrives and decorate the nursery.

Chapter 10

Sex During Pregnancy

While this book can be handy to have with you, *it should never replace the advice given by your midwife or doctor*. There are so many issues to think about while pregnant and one common question often arises 'is it safe to have sex while pregnant?' The answer is yes, if you've had a healthy pregnancy. The plug of mucus that seals your cervix, protects your baby from infection and the amniotic sac and strong uterine muscles also protect them. The baby can't tell what is going on, and don't worry your partner's penis can't penetrate beyond your vagina!

With that stated, always practice safe sex, if necessary. Just because you can't get pregnant, you can get genital herpes, STDS, etc.

However, now may not be the time to try new, crazy sex positions and even some of your favorite sex positions may not work well for you during pregnancy. A good sex position that allows you and your partner to feel good is with you on top, so no pressure goes on your bump. The following is a list of other sex positions that are comfortable: Side sex from behind, man on top (pillow under your back to lift you up). Once your baby bump starts to appear, it is important to remember not to apply pressure on it. After giving birth, sex should be put on hold until your doctor gives you the ok, typically after your six-week postnatal check. Sex can still be pleasurable during pregnancy, for both you and your partner, you just need to find out what works best for you both.

Oral sex is also fine, both if you are giving or receiving, but please make sure your partner does not blow air into your vagina. In rare cases, it can cause an air bubble (embolus) in your blood stream, which is a life-threatening condition for you and your baby.

Chapter 11

High Risk Pregnancy

High-risk pregnancy is when a condition puts the mother, baby or both at a higher risk. You are more likely to have a high-risk pregnancy if you:

- Are overweight (especially if it is by more than 22kg);
- Smoke;
- Have seizures;
- Have diabetes;
- Use drugs or alcohol;
- Are younger than 18 or older than 35;
- Have a history of genetic defects or
- You are having twins/triplets etc.

Just because you have these factors will not automatically mean you have a high-risk pregnancy and the opposite is true, just because you have no pre-existing health issues will not guarantee a healthy pregnancy. You are also at more risk if you have had any of the above issues/complications in a previous pregnancy.

If you have a pre-existing condition, you need do discuss the pros and cons of pregnancy with your GP and/or supervising consultant. There are many variables to consider and you need an expert to advise you.

Smoking Complications:

The nicotine present in cigarettes can stunt your baby's growth, and even a few cigarettes a day means harmful chemicals are reaching your baby. Smoking throughout your pregnancy can cause your baby to have a low birth weight or you may go into premature labour. You are more at risk of suffering a miscarriage, and smoking causes problems with the placenta. Babies are more likely to be ill following delivery; stay longer in hospital or even need care in the special care baby unit.

In addition, smoking during pregnancy and after your baby's birth, puts them at a higher risk of 'Sudden Infant Death Syndrome' (SIDS). Stopping smoking prior to birth is the only safe option for your baby. As soon as you give up, the baby will receive more oxygen.

NB: If you are planning a pregnancy or are pregnant and finding it hard to stop smoking, talk to your doctor about places you can get support

Alcohol:

Experts are unsure what is a safe amount of alcohol for pregnant women to drink, so if you are planning a pregnancy, or already pregnant the best advice is to abstain completely. Alcohol is passed from mother to baby, via the placenta, and it can damage and effect the cell growth of the baby (brain cells and spinal cord cells are usually the worst affected). It can cause 'Foetal Alcohol Spectrum Disorders' or the more severe 'Foetal Alcohol Syndrome'. These cause a wide range of behavioral, learning and physical problems, which can vary from mild to severe. If you are having trouble quitting alcohol, talk to your GP, so they can provide the necessary support.

Hyperemesis Gravidarum (HG):

This condition affects about 1% of pregnant women and is an excessive form of nausea and vomiting. It is not known why some women get it and others don't but some evidence shows it runs in families; and if you experienced HG in a previous pregnancy you are more likely to get it in subsequent ones. Some tips to help alleviate symptoms are:

- Rest;
- Staying hydrated;
- Avoiding nausea triggers;
- Emotional and physical support.

Not all tips work for all women, and it can be a case of trial and error to find the ones that work for you.

Be that as it may, there are medications that can help, including in the early stages of pregnancy e.g. anti-sickness drugs, steroids and vitamins B6 & B12

NB: If you are unable to keep down food and fluids contact your doctor, as you can become dehydrated very quickly when suffering with HG, and you may need to be admitted to hospital for intravenous fluid therapy.

Gestational Diabetes:

This is caused because the placenta produces hormones that lead to an increase of sugar in your blood. Your pancreas normally produces enough insulin to control this. If not, then it will cause your blood sugar to rise, and you will develop gestational diabetes. Symptoms may not necessarily arise, but can include: feeling tired; being very thirsty; weeing a lot; a dry mouth; infections like thrush, or blurred vision. Please make an appointment to see your health professional, so you can be monitored more closely. Gestational diabetes may mean you go into premature labour, so your baby will be monitored to make sure they do not show any signs of distress. After birth your baby may need to have blood tests regularly, as they may have low-blood sugar, while they adapt to making the right amount of insulin.

Pre-eclampsia:

This affects some women, usually in the second half of their pregnancy, and can even happen after their baby is born. When you see your midwife, they will monitor your blood pressure, and test a urine sample. Pre-eclampsia is one of the things they are checking for. Early signs are high blood pressure and protein found in your urine. Other symptoms include excess swelling of the hands, feet, and legs; severe headaches; vision issues. If you notice any of these symptoms, you need to seek the advice of your midwife or GP immediately. In most cases pre-eclampsia does not cause any problems, and it improves after delivery.

NB: There is a risk that pre-eclampsia can become 'eclampsia'. These are seizures, that can put both the mother and baby at risk. Contact your GP if you have any concerns.

Ectopic Pregnancy:
An ectopic pregnancy can occur when the fertilized egg implants outside of the uterus, usually in the fallopian tube. Symptoms to look out for are:

- A missed period (some women may not know they are pregnant)
- Vaginal bleeding
- Pain in your lower abdomen – on one side;
- Pain in the tip of your shoulder (no one is sure why this occurs);
- Discomfort weeing or peeing.

An ectopic pregnancy may grow large enough that it causes a fallopian tube to rupture. This is an emergency and you need surgery to repair or remove the fallopian tube. Signs of a rupture are: feeling very dizzy or faint; nausea or vomiting; looking very pale; a sharp, sudden, acute pain in your tummy. Seek medical help immediately.

Placenta Previa:
This is where the placenta lies unusually low in the uterus, and it may be near or over the surface of the cervix. Early in pregnancy it does not cause a problem, but later it can be an issue, as it will block your baby's way out. They will record the position of your placenta when you have your second scan, and if you are found to have placenta previa they will perform another scan at around the 32-week

mark. If the placenta is low it puts you at higher risk of bleeding throughout your pregnancy and labour, and this bleeding may be heavy, which puts you and your baby at risk. Your consultant may recommend that you are admitted to hospital towards the end of your pregnancy, so they can monitor you closely and emergency treatment is at hand. They will recommend you have a caesarian if the placenta is completely blocking your cervix.

NB: If you experience bright red (painless) bleeding during the last few months of pregnancy contact your midwife or doctor immediately.

Placental Abruption:
If a placental tear occurs you may notice vaginal bleeding and should seek medical attention. However, approximately 90% of these tears can heal themselves but they may also put you at an increased risk of a miscarriage, premature labour or placental abruption. This is a complication of pregnancy that means the placenta has separated from the wall of the uterus. It can deprive your baby of oxygen and nutrients but also cause severe bleeding that could be dangerous to you both.

NB: if you notice any of the following: vaginal bleeding, abdominal pain, rapid contractions, or your 'baby bump' is tender seek medical attention immediately.

Premature Labour:
Premature labour can be divided in groups:

- Extremely premature: under 28 week's gestation

- Very premature: 28 to 32 weeks

- Late prematurity: 32 to 37 weeks

Although it is important a baby gets as close to the due date as possible, sometimes things happen that are outside your control. Some factors mean you may be more at risk of premature labour. These are:

- Multiple pregnancy;

- Lifestyle factors (smoking, recreational drugs, high caffeine intake; poor diet/being underweight);

- Maternal age (under 20, over 35)

- Infections (chlamydia, untreated bladder infection);

- Cervical incompetence (the cervix opens too soon and labour follows).

While some of these cannot be avoided, others can. It is important to receive good antenatal care, have regular checkups and maintain a healthy lifestyle. If you are concerned, contact your GP/midwife immediately.

Social Factors

Older mums
You may hear the term elderly primigravida. This is from the age of 35, so not that old really, but pregnancy from this age may come with additional risks.

Most older mum's these days have chosen to delay pregnancy. Although some women have medical reasons e.g. repeated miscarriages, fertility issues. Many older mum's have chosen to delay pregnancy for social/personal reasons and they tend to be better educated, more confident and financially stable. You do however need to be aware of associated risks, some of which are:

- Decreased fertility;
- Chromosomal abnormalities;
- Developing high blood pressure or diabetes;
- Multiple births;
- Birth intervention (labour induction, forceps);
- Caesarian section.

N.B: It is best to talk to your doctor, before trying to conceive. They can give you a thorough checkup, and advice to ensure you are in good general health, and refer you to a specialist if you have any specific issues that need addressing.

Teen Pregnancy

Most girls usually start their periods about the age of 12, and teen pregnancy is defined as occurring between the age of 13 and 19 years. Teens (both girls and boys) need to be educated to realise that girls can become pregnant as soon as they begin to ovulate, so they need to practice safe sex, if they are to avoid becoming pregnant. If you are a teenager, pregnant and reading this please talk to an adult you trust: mum or dad; school counsellor/teacher, or call a support helpline. Above all you need to get help/advice and medical support for you and your baby, whether you choose to continue with the pregnancy or not.

Bed Rest

For some pregnant woman, they are advised to stay on bed rest (for a short or extended period). They may be at risk of complications such as high blood pressure; pre-eclampsia; vaginal bleeding (placenta previa, placental abruption); premature labour; threatened miscarriage; cervical insufficiency, or there may be growth issues with the baby. Some women may need to reduce their activity, or reduce their stress levels and being put on bed rest is a way to reduce unnecessary physical activities. However, being put on bed rest is not without its own issues. You may be more likely to experience heartburn, constipation, or you may just feel down as your lifestyle is curtailed. If you do find yourself feeling down, or think you me be becoming depressed, make sure to talk to your GP, as soon as possible. Also, ask friends and family to rally round and create a rota to visit you. Just remember to not overdo things!

Chapter 12

What Do I Need to Take Into Hospital?

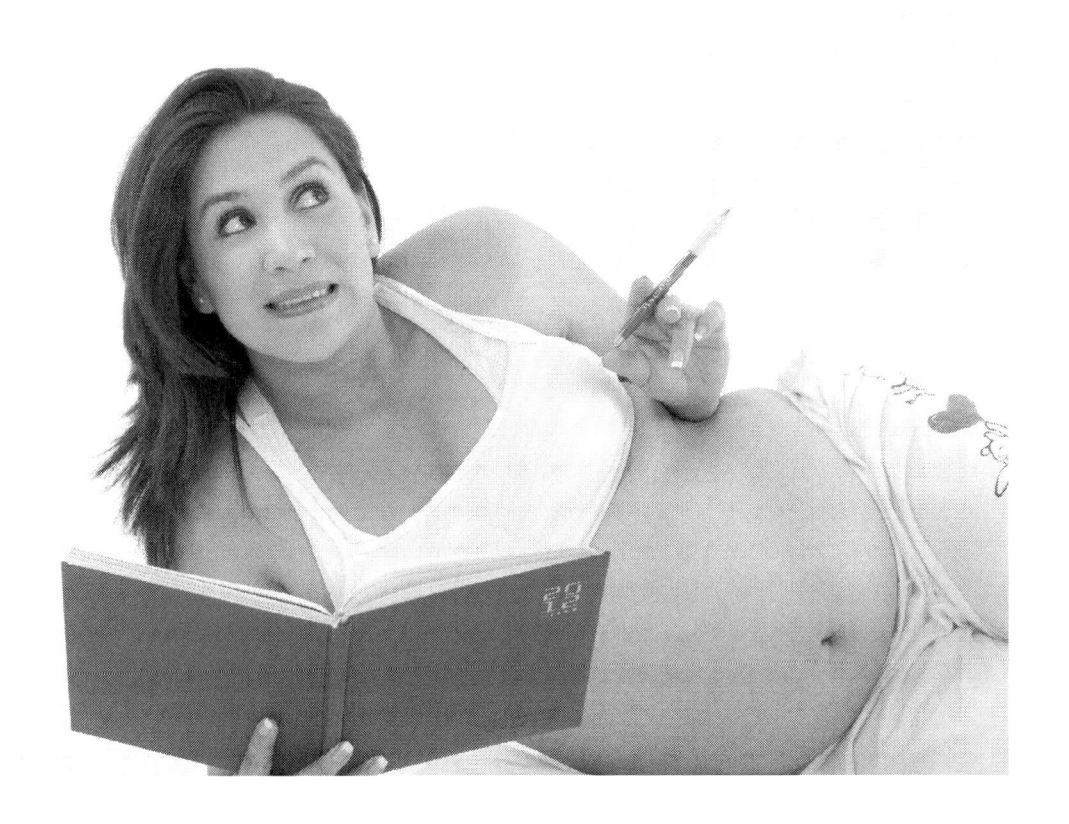

What goes in a hospital bag and when should I get it ready? Regardless of whether you are having a home, hospital or midwifery-unit birth you need to pack a bag, so everything is in one place and in case of emergencies, at least two weeks before your due date. Your midwife will provide you with a list tailored to your specific hospital/midwifery unit, but here are some things that you might want to include.

- Your birth plan, if you have written one.

- Medication/List of medication for any pre-existing conditions/illnesses you may have.
- Things to help you relax, or pass the time (music, magazines).
- Loose and comfy clothing to wear during labour. Natural fibres are a better choice, than man-made, as they let your body breathe more. You will probably need a few changes throughout labour, so make sure to pack about 3 sets. Some women may prefer to be naked throughout labour, but it is probably wise to pack them just in case. Don't forget to pack a comfortable outfit to wear home!
- About 24 extra-absorbent sanitary pads (Maternity ones with wings are a good idea).
- Sponge/cloth or a water-spray, to help keep you cool during labour.
- Front-opening, or loose-fitting nighty or tops for breastfeeding; 2 or 3 supportive but comfortable bras (make sure to take nursing bras if you are breastfeeding);
- Breast pads.
- At least 5 or 6 pairs of pants.
- Toiletry Bag;
- Towels.
- Dressing gown and slippers
- Clothing (make sure you include a hat) and nappies for the baby.
- A shawl to wrap the baby in.

- A camera to capture those all-important first moments.

Think about getting to and from the hospital, and make sure you have a contingency plan, in case of unexpected problems with transport. Think about the route you will take, to allow for unforeseen holdups e.g. roadworks. Remember, you can always call an ambulance!

NB: make sure you have rear-facing car seat (and you disable any associated air-bags). Please get expert advice, and ensure you are aware of the new, car seat regulations, that come into effect on 1st March 2017.

If you are having a home birth, you will need to discuss this with your midwife, to ensure you have everything required. But at the very least you will need clean linen and towels available for the midwife to use, sanitary pads and clothing for when your baby arrives. You also need to think about where in the home you want to give birth and if you need to hire specialist equipment e.g. a birthing pool.

Many people have mobile phones, but it can be handy to keep a written list of important contact details: Your hospital and midwife phone numbers; your partner/birth partner's phone number; your hospital reference number, as they will ask for this when you phone to say you are on your way.

Home Equipment Considerations

Babies require a lot of attention and come with a lot of baggage, literally! You may be thinking where do I start, as there are many items to buy before your baby is born. If this is your first baby you may want to buy everything in sight, but just be aware you may find you don't need it all straight away. You will find family and friends will want to help…let them!

Below is a list of items you may need immediately:
- Moses basket and stand
- Sheets and waffle blanket
- Changing table
- Baby monitor
- Baby bouncer
- Pram
- Breast feeding pillow (if required)
- Sterilizer and bottles
- Baby formula (if bottle feeding)
- A baby bath
- Nappy bag
- Scented nappy sacs

Possible purchases are:
- Bottle warmer (a jug of hot water will suffice)
- Breast pump
- Nappy bucket (for terry nappies to be collected by an agency)

- Nappy disposal Bin (these are specialist bins that lock odours away!)
- Dummies (if you think you want your baby to have one)

These things can wait to be purchased later:
- Cot
- High chair
- Safety gate and catches
- Buggy

Newborns need a lot of attention. Make sure you gather a supply of necessary equipment a couple of weeks before your due date.

Some of the obvious items your baby will need are:
- Nappies (terry or disposable);
- Baby wipes;
- Baby powder,
- Nappy rash ointment/cream,
- Baby oil/lotion,
- Baby shampoo.

Less obvious items are:
- Nail scissors (specifically for newborns);
- Baby brush;
- Baby thermometer;
- Laundry powder that is hypoallergenic,

- Thermometer for your bathtub (many parent use the elbow in the water technique, satisfactorily), *but whatever you use, be sure to put the cold water in to the bath first then the hot.* This way you avoid the possible risk of burns to the baby,

During the first weeks after your baby's arrival you may not leave the house often to buy all the necessary items, so make sure you accept help when offered. Babies go through tons of nappies but do not overstock, as they change size frequently. If you chose not to breastfeed or cannot, you will need to buy formula milk.

NB: Do not make up bottles with water straight from the tap. It needs to be freshly boiled and left to cool, for no more than 30 minutes before you make up the milk.

You are going to want to buy clothes for your baby but please remember many people may gift you baby clothes. An item you might want to buy is a swaddle blanket, this keeps your baby warm and comfortable after they are born.

Other items to buy include:
- Baby-grows/onesies;
- Socks;
- No-scratch mittens;
- Leggings,
- T-shirts,

- Cardigans/jumpers;
- Coats;
- Hats;
- Bibs;
- Burp cloths/muslins.

Keep in mind that depending when your baby is born, weather plays a factor when deciding which clothes to buy. Babies grow fast so there is no need to buy too many clothes, before they are born.

It's not just your baby that needs things ready at home for after the birth, you will too. Some items are: Nursing bras; breast pads; sanitary pads; nipple cream; comfy clothing; a supply of nutritious snacks and foods. Yet again, if people offer to cook for you, take them up on the offer! You will more than likely be able to reciprocate one day.

Refresher

Pregnancy Q & A's

We have covered some of the following, in more detail, in previous chapters. Think of these as a quick reference!

1. How do I know if I am ready to get pregnant?

Thinking about if you are ready or not is a big step. When you are properly prepared, then you will be less stressed about what could or could not happen. Before you get pregnant, it is best that you got to your OB/GYN and get a checkup as well as ask any questions that you may have about childbirth and being pregnant. During this checkup, your doctor will switch you off any medications that you may be on that could harm your fetus when you become pregnant. Moreover, they will also give you the information you need when it comes to folic acid, prenatal vitamins, and everything that you need to have or know about in order to prepare your body for conception.

2. How do I know when is the right time for me to get pregnant?

The best time for you to get pregnant is when you are ovulating. Ovulation happens typically *fourteen days* before your next period is set to start (if you are on a regular schedule. This can be difficult to track if your periods are not regular). Most cycles last twenty-four to thirty days and you will begin to ovulate somewhere between day ten and day sixteen.

3. What are the pros and cons of getting pregnant?

Everyone looks at pregnancy differently, so there are going to be different pros and cons for every woman depending on how they look at being pregnant.

A few cons that are quite common amongst mothers are:

- The decisions that you have to make with regards to getting prenatal screenings, what you are going to do with the results, so on and so forth.

- The lack of alcohol. You are not supposed to drink while you are pregnant. Even though some doctors will tell you that it is okay for you to have a glass or two in moderation, there are others who will tell you to stay away from it completely. It is up to you on whether or not you heed their warning.

- How pregnancy is going to affect your body. Yes, your body is going to change because you are having a child that is growing in your womb thus making not only your abdomen extend as they get bigger, but changing things such as how your breasts appear and things like that.

- Mood swings and lack of sleep. Thanks to the amount of hormones that are flooding your system, you may find that you are more irritable at times than others and that you are having problems sleeping when your baby actually gets here.

Some pros are:

- Bigger breasts. As you go through your pregnancy, your breasts are going to grow large due to the milk that is being produced in preparation for the breast feeding process.

- Being spoiled with love and care. Many women experience that their partners, their friends, and their families tend to spoil them when they find out that they are pregnant because everyone is excited for the baby!

- Your hair and nails are going to grow faster thanks to all those hormones (they are not all bad, they just tend to get a little bit irritating when it comes to certain aspects of your pregnancy).

4. What is the food I cannot eat during pregnancy?

It is suggested that you need to stay away from:

- Fish that contains a lot of mercury. Having large amounts of mercury in your system can actually end up damaging a developing brain.
- You should also stay away from any unpasteurized soft cheeses such as brie, feta, gorgonzola, etc.
- Raw fish such as sushi.
- Cold ready to eat meals like hot dogs or lunch meat because of the listeria that the meat can contain.
- Unpasteurized milk (which is also a source of listeria).

- Alcohol due to the fact that it can interfere with the development of your fetus and even lead to fetal alcohol syndrome.

- Uncooked or cured eggs and meats such as prosciutto, or runny eggs.

- Caffeine however it is okay when you take it in moderate amounts.

5. What foods should I eat while I am pregnant?

Above all you need to follow a healthy diet and your body needs extra vitamins and minerals. Whatever anybody may tell you, you do not need to 'eat for two'. It is advised that you eat an extra 350 to 500 calories (1470 to 2090 kilo-joules) during the 2nd and 3rd trimesters. If your diet is lacking, it may affect the baby's development.

Poor eating habits and gaining excess weight can put you at a higher risk of gestational diabetes, or birth complications. Things such as leafy greens, vegetables, fruits, whole grain breads and cereals are going to be the best option, while you are pregnant. You also need to consume food that contain protein and calcium, such as low fat yogurts, broccoli, eggs, salmon. When it comes to meat, please refer to the section on what not to eat, but above all make sure the meat is cooked thoroughly!

6. Does it matter if I miss a day of my pregnancy vitamins?

Prenatal vitamins are important in helping to bridge the gap in any of the nutrients that you may be missing in your diet. However, if you happen to miss a day or two of your prenatal vitamins, you are not going to find that anything is going to happen to you or your baby. There are some women who never take prenatal vitamins when they are pregnant.

7. What should I do if I become constipated during pregnancy?

Constipation is something that many pregnant women complain about. This is not too uncommon for women during some point in their pregnancy. With all the progesterone in your system, you are going to realize that your muscles are smoothed out and relaxed, and this also affects the digestive tract.

Due to all the progesterone, your food is going to pass through your digestive system slower. Not only that, but taking iron supplements in high doses is going to cause you to have constipation.

In order to combat constipation, you can:

(a) Drink plenty of water

Your urine should look clear. One glass of juice a day will help as well, most particularly prune juice in order to help regulate your digestive system. There have been reports that drinking some sort of warm liquid after you get up will also help to keep you from being constipated.

(b) Eat foods that are high in fiber

This should be things such as whole grain breads and cereals along with brown rice, beans, and fresh vegetables and fruits. You can also include a tablespoon or two of unprocessed wheat bran with your breakfast along with a glass of water to help you get things moving.

(c) Look at your prenatal vitamins

If they contain a high amount of iron, then ask your healthcare provider about switching to a different prenatal that does not have so much iron in it. The only reason that you need a lot of iron is because you are anemic and are needing to increase your iron intake.

(d) Exercise regularly

Doing light exercises such as swimming, yoga, riding a stationary bike, or even walking can help you to ease the pain of constipation and leave you not only feeling better, but feeling healthier.

(e) After you eat, use the bathroom.

Your body knows when you need to get rid of the waste in it; so listen to it. Do not put off going to the bathroom once you feel the need to. Doing this can cause problems later on.

If all else fails, talk to your doctor about prescribing you something that can help or about adding an over the counter fiber supplement or even stool softener to your daily routine.

The only time that you should begin to worry about your constipation is if there are other symptoms with it such as, abdominal pain, you are passing mucus or blood, or you are having constipation and then diarrhea alternating. At this point in time, you need to get in contact with your doctor or other health care provider as it may be a different issue that is causing this.

While you are going to the bathroom, try not to strain. If you strain you can end up causing hemorrhoids or even cause them to worsen if you already have them. This is caused by the swelling of the veins in your rectal area.

Hemorrhoids are painful and uncomfortable, but will end up going away when you give birth to your baby. If you find that the pain is too severe or you are having bleeding from your rectal, you need to call your health care provider to see if there is a more serious issue going on.

8. What exercises can I do while I am pregnant?

While you are pregnant, you are able to do activities such as swimming, walking, a stationary bike, low impact aerobics, a step machine, and even an elliptical machine. You can also do things such as tennis, racquetball and jogging.

However, you need to be careful and talk to your health care provider if you are unsure if you should be doing the activity.

9. What are my exercise limitations while I am pregnant?

Most exercises you are going to be able to do and you are probably going to slow down and change your routines as your abdomen gets bigger. However, you are going to want to avoid things that are going to give you a higher risk of falling or any kind of abdominal injury.

Along with those, you are going to want to avoid any high altitude sports.

10. Can I have sex while I am pregnant?

Yes!

If your partner is scared of having intercourse with you while you are pregnant. Reassure him that he is not going to hurt you or the baby. If he is still unsure about it, then talk to your doctor about ways that you can help calm his fears so you can get back to doing what you want to do.

11. What is first trimester screening?

This is a test that is done early in your pregnancy in order to offer some information about the chromosomal risks for things such as Down syndrome. Testing is done by either a blood test or by an ultrasound exam.

12. What do I do with my first trimester screening results?

Your results are going to tell you if your baby is at risk for Down syndrome. This test does not mean that your child will have Down syndrome, it only tells you the risk of carrying a baby with this genetic condition.

13. What symptoms are normal while I am pregnant?

There are different symptoms that you will experience while you are pregnant, however, some of the symptoms you may experience are:

- Swelling and bloating,
- Acne,
- Cramping,
- Changes in your sleep pattern,
- Sensitivities

14. Is it normal to have extra discharge while pregnant?

Yes. Not only are your hormones sky-rocketing due to your baby, you also have extra blood flow going to your pelvis. There is a high possibility that you are going to notice an increase in discharge as you go through your pregnancy.

If you find that your discharge has a color, an odor, is painful, or is watery, you need to contact your doctor right away. This could mean that you have an infection of some sort that needs to be treated, or even that your water has broken.

15. What can I expect from my emotions?

You can expect your emotions to be all over the place thanks to the hormones that you have in your system. You may feel like laughing one minute and crying the next. This is perfectly normal.

16. How much is your baby growing each month?

Month one:

This is going to be when your embryo is still starting to develop. There are going to be two layers of cells that are going to help to develop all the organs and vital body parts that your baby is going to need in order to survive.

Month two:

At this point, your little one is the size of a kidney bean and will be moving. There will be webbed fingers, but you can very distinctly see that he or she actually has fingers!

Month three:

During this month your baby is going to be around three inches long and is going to have the same weight as a pea pod. Not only that, but his fingerprints have now developed making him his own unique person!

Month four:

Your baby is now about 5.5 inches long and weighs somewhere around five ounces. It is during this month that he is going to begin to have his skeleton harden from the cartilage that makes up our skeleton to the bones that are going to help him hold his shape and move around.

Month five:

Ten and a half inches in length, your baby now has eyelids and eyebrows. He is also able to stretch out his legs (this is where you will probably begin to feel more kicks).

Month six:

The wrinkles on your baby's skin are starting to smooth out as he begins to put on more weight. With that weight gain, your baby now weighs around a pound and a half.

Month seven:

Your baby can now see what is around him and can open and close his eyes. Your baby is also one and a half inches long.

Month eight:

As baby fills out to be rounder and more fully developed, your baby now weights around 4.7 pounds. Not only that, but his lungs are now developed and he is able to breath better.

Month nine:

You're now ready for your baby to come any day now! Baby is around twenty and a half inches long and weighs about seven and a half pounds (could be larger, could be smaller). However, your baby is fully developed and ready to be held by you!

17. Why am I always tired?

During the early and late stages of your pregnancy, you may realize that you are more tired because your hormones are working overtime in order to keep up with all the changes that your body is making for both you and the baby.

It is also possible that you are having trouble sleeping at night because of things like having to go pee all the time, heartburn, or even leg cramps.

18. Will my frequent urination stop while I am pregnant?

Your constant need to urinate will ease up after your baby is born. In the days immediately following the baby's birth, you may realize that you are urinating more often because your body is attempting to get rid of all the fluids that your body retained while you were pregnant.

19. Why am I experiencing headaches while I am pregnant?

You may be experiencing headaches that range from mild to intense due to the rise in hormone production. This is your body's way of trying to accommodate the sudden rises in hormones.

Once your body is used to the hormones, your headache should ease up. If they do not, it is best that you talk to your health care provider.

20. Does being pregnant really cause lower back pain?

Yes, pregnancy really does cause lower back pain. This is usually caused because your center of gravity has shifted to the front of your body due to your ever-growing abdomen.

Changing the way that you sit and sleep can help to ease some of the back pain that you are feeling. If you sleep on your side, you may want to place a pillow between your knees.

You may feel an increase in back pain right before you go into labor.

21. How do I treat morning sickness?

It's an unpleasant side effect but your baby is not at increased risk. Most women find it starts to clear up by week 16 to 20. The following may help to reduce the symptoms, sometimes it is a case of trial and error.

- Get plenty of rest: tiredness can increase nausea.
- Ensure you drink plenty of water, to stay hydrated, but sip fluid. Little and often is better than one large drink, you may find you vomit otherwise. Drinks that are very sharp, sweet or too cold can make nausea or sickness worse.
- If you are feeling sick when you wake up, make sure you take your time getting out of bed. If you can, have something to eat prior to doing so e.g. a dry biscuit, toast.

- Eat smaller meals, more regularly. Foods that are high in carbohydrate can help e.g. pasta, bread, crackers. Pregnant women often find savoury foods are tolerated better than spicy or sweet ones. **NB:** Don't stop eating! If you find the nausea and vomiting prevents you eating, you must consult your healthcare professional.

- Avoid smells or foods that make you feel sick. Some women find they prefer eating cold meals to hot ones, as they don't give off as much aroma. Ask someone else to do the cooking. If this is not an option, try to cook bland foods, like pasta, that don't give off too much of a smell and are easy to prepare.

- Sometimes the more you think about nausea the worse it can be, so try to find something distracting to do. Adjusting the clothing you wear can also help. Trade in your tight jeans for ones with a comfortable elastic waistband

- You may find that ginger products help to counteract nausea, but they are not licensed in the UK. Make sure you buy them from a reputable source, like a pharmacy. You might find that ginger biscuits or ginger ale help.

22. How do I know what trimester I am in?

Your first trimester is going to be months one through three. Otherwise known as week zero to week thirteen. The second trimester is week fourteen to week twenty-seven months four to seven. Month seven to nine is the third trimester. This is week twenty-eight to when you give birth.

23. How much weight should I gain while pregnant?

Normal weight gain for a pregnant woman is twenty-five to thirty-five pounds.

Should you be overweight, your weight gain is supposed to be around fifteen to twenty-five pounds.

If you are underweight then it is safe for you to gain twenty-eight to forty pounds.

If you are having multiple births, you should only gain about thirty-five to forty-five pounds.

24. Is gas and indigestion normal while pregnant?

Yes. With the changes in hormones, the efficiency of the gastrointestinal system is lowered. The first sign is going to probably be nausea and morning sickness. As your pregnancy progresses, it can change into acid reflux and indigestion. This is completely normal.

25. When will my morning sickness end?

For most women morning sickness stops at twelve weeks. However, some women end up having morning sickness till the end of their pregnancy.

Morning sickness is not harmful to your or your fetus. It is only harmful if you begin to experience excessive vomiting and find that you are not able to manage to keep your food down.

26. What are activities I should avoid while I am pregnant?

You do not want to change the cat box. Doing this task can actually end up leading to complications for newborns.

- Paint. The exposure to the toxic chemicals is not good for you or baby.

- Get an X-Ray unless you absolutely have to.

- Use a sauna, hot tub or tanning booth.

- Go on rides such as Great American Scream Machine or Tower of Terror.

27. What can I do to relieve or prevent heartburn?

In order to prevent heartburn, you should try and avoid greasy and spicy foods as well as drinks that contain a lot of caffeine. You can also try and eat smaller meals while avoiding having to bend or lay down right after you have eaten.

28. What can I do to relieve or prevent leg cramps?

Make sure that you exercise regularly and are getting plenty of fluids in your system. It is also important that you do not sit in one position for an extended period of time. Massage your legs in order to keep blood flowing and apply heat when you need to relieve a cramp.

29. What can I do to relieve or prevent hemorrhoids?

Drink plenty of fluids and make sure that you have plenty of fiber in your diet. Exercising regularly and avoiding standing or sitting for long periods of time.

You can also try and take sitz baths while applying cold compresses to the effect area.

30. What are some of the complications that I can experience while pregnant?

(a) Before Pregnancy:

As you are trying to get pregnant, you need to make sure you talk to your health care provider about any health issues you currently going through or have experienced in order to make sure they do not cause any complications later in your pregnancy.

If the issue is current, then it may require you to change how you and your doctor are treating that issue due to the medication possibly causing an issue later on.

Also, it is important that you identify any issues that you had in previous pregnancies in order to try and get them addressed and possibly avoid them with this pregnancy.

(b) During Pregnancy:

While pregnant, the complications and even the symptoms of these complications can range anywhere from annoying and slightly uncomfortable all the way to something that can be life-threatening.

Not all the symptoms are going to be physical either. There are some mental issues that the mother can have that can end up effecting not only the mother, but the baby as well.

It is vitally important that you keep track of these symptoms and if anything troubling happens or begins to worry you, talk to your health care provider in an effort to try and prevent any further issues.

(c) Pregnancy Complications:

Urinary Tract Infection (UTI): this is a bacterial infection that occurs in your urinary tract. Signs that you have a UTI are:

- Nausea or back pain
- Fever, tiredness, shakiness
- Pressure in your lower stomach
- Urine that smells bad or looks cloudy or reddish
- An urge to use the bathroom often
- Pain or a burning sensation when you use the bathroom.

Should you believe that you have a UTI, it is important that you talk to your doctor about being tested. If you test positive, then your doctor will be able to give you a treatment of antibiotics so that you can kill the infections to make it better in a day or two.

(d) Anemia:

This is when there is a lower number of red blood cells than what you should have in your body. When you are being treated for the underlying cause of anemia, then you will be able to restore the number of healthy red blood cells. There is a possibility that you will feel tired as well as weak should you have anemia. This can be treated by taking folic acid and even iron supplements.

(e) Mental Health Conditions:

You may even experience depression while you are pregnant. If your depression persists throughout your entire pregnancy, you may want to consider talking to a therapist in order to help you get your depression treated. Depression can actually end up causing you to have trouble taking care of your baby after they are born.

A few other complications that you may come across are, obesity and weight gain, infections, high blood pressure, hyperemesis gravidarum (morning sickness/nausea), or GDM (Gestational Diabetes Mellitus).

31. Is bleeding cause for alarm while I am pregnant?

Yes! Bleeding can actually mean that there are complications occurring in your pregnancy and you need to be seen immediately.

Anything from zero to twenty weeks means that you could be having a miscarriage.

Anything between twenty to thirty-seven weeks means that you could be having preterm labor

And at any time it could mean that there are problems with your placenta such as it having separated from the inner wall of your uterus.

32. How bad will my pregnancy dizziness get?

It is a common symptom to feel dizzy while you are pregnant. During your early pregnancy it means that you could have low blood sugar and need to eat something. You may feel dizzy up until you give birth due to your uterus putting pressure on the arteries in your legs. However, always try and eat something to make sure it is not just low blood sugar.

33. How will I know if I am in labor?

You will know you are in labor when you begin to experience

- Strong contractions that are happening at short intervals,
- Your water has broken,
- You are having cramps in your lower back that are not going away,
- You have a blood mucus discharge.

34. How do I know when I am ready to push?

You will push when you are experiencing a contraction after you have fully dilated. Your nurse or doctor will keep track of how far dilated you are and will tell you when it is safe for you to push and when it is not. You will not push when you are not having a contraction because that will just cause your labor to be harder than necessary.

35. How do I know if the time is right to become pregnant?
Having a baby is a big step. If you are properly prepared, then you will find you will be less stressed whilst trying to conceive and during pregnancy. As they say, 'forewarned is forearmed'. Before you try to conceive, it is best to schedule an appointment with your doctor. They can carry out a general health check and it is a chance for you and your partner to ask questions you may have, about pregnancy and childbirth. If you are on any regular medication or have a chronic illness, this is the time to discuss the issue with your doctor and they can arrange for you to see a consultant. Moreover, your doctor can provide you with information in regards to folic acid, antenatal vitamins, and other steps to prepare your body for conception.

36. What other considerations are there before I have a baby?
Every woman looks at pregnancy differently, therefore there will be very individual considerations/reactions. Some women seem to breeze through pregnancy. Others, can experience quite negative feelings, and this can be quite normal. It is a big step to take and there is a lot to consider. Are you going to undergo antenatal screening? If you do and you receive unwelcome results, how are you going to react/what is your next step?

37. What to do if nausea and vomiting become more severe?

If your nausea and vomiting becomes severe and does not respond to the remedies above, you might find your GP prescribes a short course of anti-sickness (antiemetic) medication. Some antihistamines (for allergies) can also help control sickness. Do not take anything unless it has been prescribed especially for you!

N.B: We discussed Hyperemesis Gravidarum in chapter 7. It needs specialist treatment in hospital, so please contact your doctor if you are concerned

38. What supplements should I take before and during pregnancy?

Folic Acid is a must as soon as you plan on becoming pregnant. You need to take 400 micrograms every day, while you are trying to conceive and up until you are 12 weeks. Why? Folic Acid can help to reduce neural tube defects, such as Spina Bifida. Obviously check with your midwife or doctor first but you need to choose an antenatal vitamin that includes: Folic acid, vitamin D, calcium, vitamin C, thiamine, riboflavin, niacin, and vitamin B12.

39. When will I start to feel the baby move?

Baby movement or 'quickening' is usually felt between weeks 16 to 25. In your first pregnancy, it might not be until closer to the 25 weeks. In a woman's second or subsequent pregnancy they may feel it at 13 weeks. Remember every woman is different but if you are at all concerned talk to your midwife or doctor.

40. What medication can I take while I am pregnant?

With any medication in pregnancy, whether supermarket or pharmacy bought you should discuss taking them with your doctor. There are some herbal/alternative remedies that are safe to take whilst pregnant to relieve things such as nausea. Some are not! So please check with your GP/midwife, before taking them. Also, make sure you adhere to the correct dose. Do not take an increased dose, thinking it will be more effective!

41. Why am I experiencing headaches, while pregnant?

In early pregnancy, there is an increase in hormones and blood flow, and this may mean more frequent headaches. Other causes can be stress, low blood sugar, tiredness and dehydration. Later in pregnancy they tend to be caused due to poor posture. Whatever the cause, before you take any medication to combat them, talk to your GP first.

N.B: Headaches in the 3rd trimester can also be caused by pre-eclampsia (discussed in chapter 7), so make sure you attend regular antenatal checkups, and if you are at all concerned contact your midwife or doctor.

42. Why am I getting lower back pain?

Your body produces a hormone (relaxin) that causes the ligaments in your pelvic area to relax. It may also cause ligaments in your spine to loosen, which can cause pain. Your spine supports the extra weight gained in pregnancy, and your growing uterus puts pressure on nerves and blood vessels in your back and pelvis. Your centre of gravity changes due to weight gain later in pregnancy, so you may start to change the way you stand/move to compensate. Trying the following may help: Regular exercise, to strengthen muscles and to improve your flexibility; improved posture (make sure you don't slouch). Changing the way, you sit and sleep can also help to ease any back pain that you are feeling. If you sleep on your side, you may want to try placing a pillow between your knees.

43. Is heartburn and indigestion common while pregnant?
Digestion is slowed down in pregnancy, due to progesterone making muscles smoother. The valve at the top of the oesophagus can also open or leak, which then lets stomach acid flow upwards. In addition, as your uterus grows, it pushes on your stomach causing more pressure on the valve. To help avoid heartburn, try not to eat greasy or spicy foods, and drinks that contain a lot of caffeine. You can also try and eat smaller meals, while avoiding bending or laying down right after you have eaten.

44. Is it normal to have extra discharge while pregnant?
Yes, but it should be thin, white and normally odourless or mild smelling, and is caused by having extra blood flow going to your pelvis. If you find the discharge changes colour, smells, looks unusual, or you experience pain, itching or soreness, contact your GP. It may mean you have thrush, and this is easily treated.

N.B: Do not use tampons whilst pregnant, as more germs may be introduced into your vagina.

45. How can I relieve leg cramps?

No one is exactly sure what causes leg cramps. But there are a few things you can do if you get them:

- Straighten your leg, then (gently) flex your toes and ankles towards your calf.
- Try standing on a cold surface, as this can sometimes stop a spasm

N.B: If the flexing or cold do not work, make sure you see you GP, immediately. In rare instances the pain could be due to a blood clot. Do not massage, as this could make it worse.

46. Can I prevent stretch marks

Stretch marks are caused, in later pregnancy due to changes in elastic tissue that is just below the skin's surface. Genetics can play a part in whether you get them or not. Although you may not be able to avoid them, you may be able to slow them down. No stretch mark cream is going to prevent them but massaging your skin, with an oil or cream can help you to feel good, and it may even encourage new tissue growth.

47. Is it safe to fly while pregnant?

If you are only having one baby, and your pregnancy has been a healthy one, then you can usually fly up until you're 36 weeks pregnant. Some airlines are reluctant to carry women after 28 weeks, due to the risk they may go into premature labour, so check with the individual airline. If you have a high-risk pregnancy, your doctor may advise you not to fly throughout your pregnancy.

48. Can I eat a vegetarian diet whilst pregnant?

Make sure you plan your meals, and eat a variety of healthy, nutritious vegetarian foods, then you should be able to continue. Make sure you consume all the necessary vitamins, minerals, protein and nutrients that you and your baby need. If in doubt, talk to your midwife or doctor.

Conclusion

Through pregnancy, your baby grows a little every day and your body is designed to change and keep them safe. During each stage, you and your baby go through many changes. With each trimester comes new discoveries and the imminent arrival of your little one can be scary, stressful but more than anything - exciting.

During pregnancy and beyond a woman's life changes forever, and hopefully this book has helped you prepare for these changes. It has covered topics such as symptoms of pregnancy, nutrition and risk factors. If you are experiencing unusual or painful symptoms, be sure to contact your midwife/doctor, immediately. If you are planning a pregnancy, hopefully this book will help you to be well prepared for the journey you may someday embark on. More than anything, enjoy your pregnancy and congratulations for that beautiful baby boy or girl!

Part II

Breastfeeding

A

Beginners Guide to **Infant Feeding**

Diapering and Circumcision

By

Dr. Jane Smart

www.MillenniumPublishingLimited.com

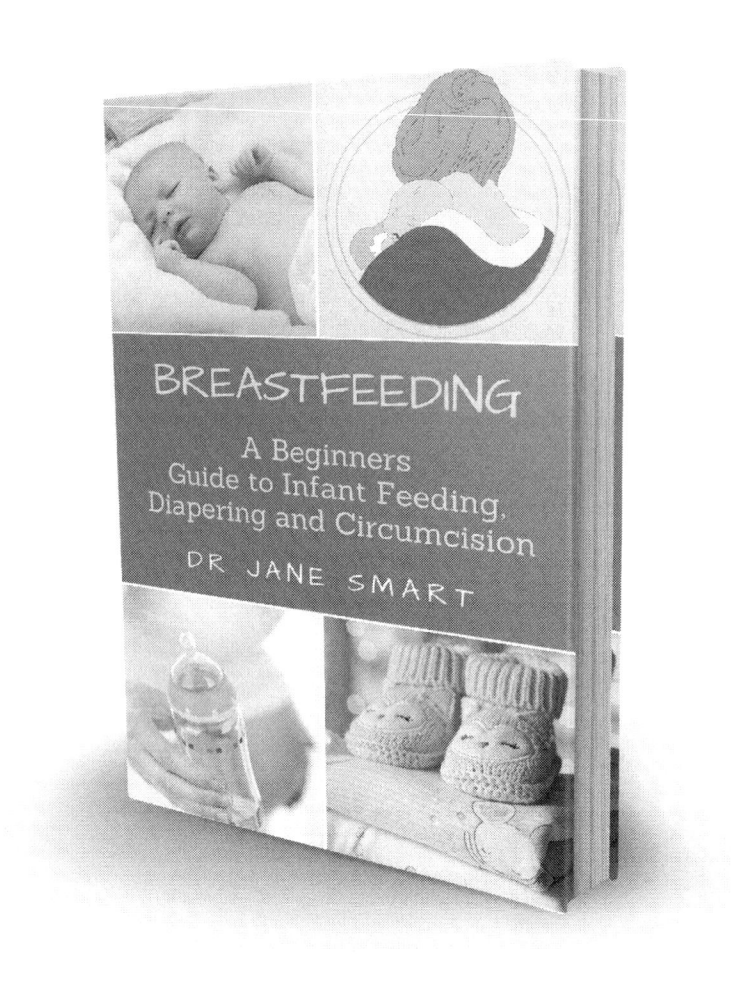

Available in kindle, Paperback and Audio format

Introduction II

Infant feeding, diapering, and circumcision are some of the first decisions you will make as a new parent. Infant feeding has complex social influences with a wide variety of factors to consider. The feeding options include exclusive breastfeeding, breast milk pumping and bottle-feeding, formula feeding, or a combination thereof. Breastfeeding has a long history of biological and emotional benefits. The alternative methods of breastfeeding have a storied history, as well.

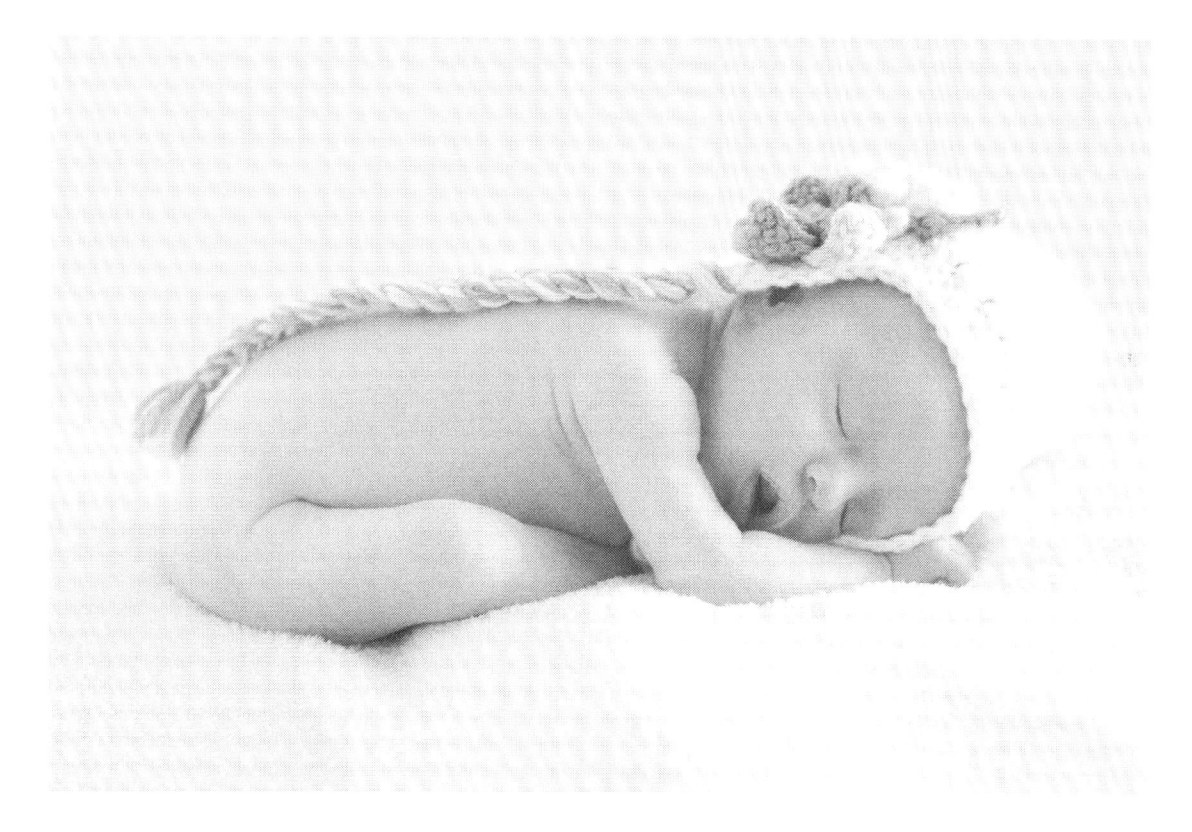

Bathing your baby is one of the first tasks that new parents experience. The newborn bath can be nerve-wracking with a slippery baby. It is important to keep your baby safe, comfortable, and warm during bath time.

Baby diapering boasts the choices of either cloth or disposable. Some families opt to use a cloth diaper service to pick up and launder the diapers, while others prefer to wash them at home. The choices are extensive if you choose to go the disposable diaper route. If you walk into any baby store, you will notice the long row of disposable diaper options on the wall.

Circumcision is a wildly controversial topic with staunch supporters on either side. This book will discuss the recommendations of the professional organizations for male circumcision, considerations, and what to expect in the process. Finally, this book will also touch on the subject of female circumcision.

Please note: this book is in no way a replacement for the professional care a doctor can provide. So please talk to them if anything is concerning you

Chapter 13

History of Infant Feeding

The evolution of feeding infants is rooted deeply in breastfeeding. However, breastfeeding has moved in and out of fashion throughout time. In Israel around 2000 BC, children were considered a blessing and breastfeeding was a religious obligation. In fact, the Bible describes wet nurses.

In one famous biblical passage, the Pharaoh's daughter, a princess, found baby Moses floating in a basket in the Nile River by the bulrushes. The princess did not have any children and brought the baby to the palace and adopted Moses. She needed a wet nurse to breastfeed him, and through a series of divine interventions, Moses own mother was hired to be his wet nurse.

In Greece around 950 BC, socialite women demanded wet nurses. They were able to afford wet nurses and enjoyed the prestige involved. Wet nurses enjoyed power and status over other slaves. The height of the Roman Empire was between 300 BC and 400 AD. Wet nurses who fed abandoned infants received employment contracts. These contracts cover the information regarding their length of service and payment amount. Rich women often employed wet nurses, as well.

In the Middle Ages, breast milk was believed to have magical qualities that transmitted the characteristics of the breastfeeding mother. Childhood was regarded as a time of helplessness and fragility. It was important for a mother to nurse her own child and considered a virtuous duty. This was a time where even the wealthy were encouraged to breastfeed their own children.

During the Renaissance period, breastfeeding mothers continue to be fashionable. In fact, mothers disapproved of wet-nursing unless absolutely necessary and had a strong preference for mothers who breastfed their own children.

In 16th and 17th century Europe, society believed that infants would come to love the wet nurse more than the mother because she had been the nurturing figure. Mothers were persuaded to nurse their own children so that their babies would take on the characteristics of their mother, rather than the wet nurse.

Aristocratic women rarely breastfed because the practice was passé and they worried they would ruin their figures. It also interfered with wearing fashionable clothing. The wives of merchants, lawyers, and doctors did not breastfeed because it was cheaper to hire a wet nurse than someone to assist with the household and family business.

In 1800, society believed that it was natural, enjoyable, and fulfilled their God-given role as mothers and nurturers. Breastfeeding was the ideal for the Victorian nuclear family life. It continued to be the preferred method of feeding for upper and middle-class families through the turn of the century.

During the 19th century, Sigmund Freud instead that infants suckles for sexual pleasure which encouraged mothers to bottle-feed. Both caused a decline in breastfeeding. At this time, America experienced a milk shortage and encouraged the dangerous practice of giving cow's milk to babies.

Cow's milk contains high concentrations of protein that cause stress on the kidneys. It worsens conditions like heat stroke, diarrhea, and fever. Cow's milk does not contain enough iron, vitamin C, and other nutrients. Babies who consumed this were at risk for rickets, scurvy, malnourishment, and bacterial infections.

In 1865, the chemist Justus von Liebig developed and sold an infant food consisting of cow's milk, flour, and potassium bicarbonate. It could be in either liquid or powder form. By 1883, there were 27 brands of infant formula.

After World War II, infant formula became in vogue. The era's top echelon mothers adopted the more fashionable bottle-feeding since the lower class could not afford it. Breastfeeding became viewed as unsanitary and old-fashioned. In the 1950s, the majority of women bottle-fed.

By the end of the 1930s, evaporated milk was used as a baby formula and its popularity surpassed all commercial formulas in the United States. By 1950, the majority of all babies were raised on evaporated milk. In response to this rate of formula and evaporated milk feeding, a group promoting breastfeeding and supporting nursing mothers started the La Leche League in the United States.

In 1956, the La Leche League wanted to appeal to new moms. They produced a pamphlet stating, "With his small head pillowed against your breast and your milk warming his insides, your baby knows a special closeness to you, he is gaining a firm foundation in an important area of life-he is learning about love."

Currently, the pendulum has swung back in the other direction. Eighty percent of all mothers initiate breastfeeding at birth. Only half of all breastfeeding mothers continue to breastfeed at six months of age. In fact, only one in four breastfeeding mothers is nursing in some capacity at twelve months. Many experts and celebrities speak out strongly in support of breastfeeding. Breastfeeding is now considered the preferred and natural method.

Chapter 14

Historical Alternatives to Breastfeeding

A wet nurse is a woman who breastfeeds another woman's child. It started as early as 2000 BC to provide nutrition for babies who were unable to be fed by their mother due to lactation issues or death during childbirth. It was considered the best alternative to the baby's biological mother's milk.

It continued as the preferred alternative method of infant feeding until the turn of the century. However, some women could not breastfeed or simply favored hiring a wet nurse. Unfortunately, wet nurses were poor black or immigrant women who were not allowed to bring their children into their employer's households. Often wet nurses' babies suffered from malnutrition and neglect, and many even died while their mothers nourished others children. This continued until the 1920s when many wet nurses were able to sell their milk to be bottled.

Ultimately, society's negative views surrounding wet nursing led to the substitution of formula and bottle-feeding. In 1910, formula bottle-feeding rose in popularity and by the 1950s, eighty percent of women bottle-fed. It was considered fashionable and modern. While breastfeeding has regained popularity, bottle-feeding retains its role as a viable and healthy option for babies.

Chapter 15

Social Pressure & infant Feeding

In our society, the decision for which type of infant feeding is preferable is difficult enough if it occurred in a vacuum. However, when faced with the social pressure to breastfeed or bottle-feed, it becomes overwhelming. Once you've made your choice, the social pressure does not always fade.

Family, friends, co-workers, and complete strangers are likely to give you their opinion on what you should be doing with your new baby and what you are doing wrong. Parenting is complicated enough without feeling that you are a failure. There are conflicting opinions on how to feed your baby, diaper your baby, and whether to circumcise. Even if you have made the decision to breastfeed, there are still other considerations like what age to stop breastfeeding, where it is appropriate to breastfeed, whether you should pump your breasts, and if you should breastfeed while juggling work and other children.

These controversial discussions are enough to make any educated mother question their choices. Unfortunately, well-meaning family members may be a barrier to bonding with your new baby. In their excitement to see their new tiny family member, they may make it difficult for you to learn the ropes of breastfeeding or have private time to nurse and to bond.

While these obstacles may seem overwhelming, knowing about these potential barriers can promote your ability to create a plan on how to best deal with them. You know your family best of all and who the offenders will be. In the case of family members who linger, do not be afraid to ask for help with chores or for privacy. Finally, discuss ahead of time with your partner if he or she is willing to be the "bad guy" to end visiting time in order to promote family bonding time when guests have left.

Most importantly, sit with your partner and make your own parenting choices. Educate yourself regarding all the options, make up your mind, and be confident with your decision. At the end of the day, the choice is between you and your baby.

Chapter 16

Breastfeeding Basics

Breastfeeding literally means to feed your baby with milk from the breast. It is a beautiful time of bonding, nourishment, and focusing on the shift in your new role as a mother. It is also a frustrating time while you learn an important new skill, worry about the health of your baby, and experience strange physical sensations and breast issues. Breastfeeding is both natural and complicated. It may require more preparation and assistance than you anticipate.

Breastfeeding initiation involves a slew of hormonal, physical, and mental changes designed to help you emotionally and physically nourish your child. The hormonal changes involve two hormones called oxytocin and prolactin. Prolactin is a hormone made in the pituitary gland in the brain in both men and women. While it has other functions, it is primarily known as the breastfeeding hormone because it is the main hormone needed for lactation. Prolactin prepares your breasts to make milk during pregnancy. The placenta creates high levels of hormones that prevent the prolactin from producing much breast milk.

After the birth of the placenta, the hormonal levels decrease which allows the prolactin to tell your breasts to make milk. The initial milk is called colostrum which is the yellow, fatty breast milk produced immediately postpartum. It takes several days, but the surge in breast milk after birth is caused by prolactin.

However, prolactin alone is not enough to continue to make breast milk. You must continue to breastfeed in order to create enough for your baby.

When you breastfeed your baby (or pump your breasts), the nerves signal your brain to release oxytocin and prolactin. Oxytocin is a hormone and neurotransmitter known as the "hormone of love". Oxytocin is made in the brain's hypothalamus and secreted by the pituitary gland, a pea-sized structure at the base of the brain.

Oxytocin is pivotal for breastfeeding because it causes the milk ejection (or let-down reflex) by stimulating the muscles surrounding the breast to squeeze out the milk. Both mom and baby release it during breastfeeding. While it plays an important role in breastfeeding, it plays a huge role in the relationship between a mom and her baby. It causes drowsiness, euphoria, increases the pain threshold, and promotes love for one another. Oxytocin magically strengthens the bond between mama and baby.

Oxytocin is an important chemical for you and your baby. It is naturally released during labor and birth to offset painful contractions by stimulating the production of chemicals that make you feel happy known as endorphins. It naturally combats painful contractions by this release of endorphins. Extraordinarily, it behaves differently in its natural form than it does in its man-made form.

Hospital labor and delivery units harness the childbirth hormone through a synthetic intravenous (IV) drip. This IV drip is known by the brand name Pitocin. It is given during labor augmentation and induction to increase uterine contraction strength, frequency, and length during labor. It is also given to prevent excessive bleeding in the postpartum period. Synthetic oxytocin has side effects that natural oxytocin does not. These include uterine rupture, rapid heartbeat, and unusual bleeding.

Natural (endogenous) oxytocin is released in short and frequent pulses, while synthetic oxytocin is continuously administered. It is also given in higher doses than occurs naturally. Synthetic oxytocin does not cross the blood-brain barrier. This means that it does not have the same effect on the brain and bonding with baby.

Beyond the labor and birth experience, oxytocin is released during snuggling, hugging, and orgasm. It influences stress regulation and mental health. Oxytocin is associated with empathy, trust, sexual activity, and relationship building. It also has social functions by impacting social bonding (pro-social and anti-social behavior), social recognition, and creating group memories.

While the hormonal effects are strong, the physical act of touching is also important. Breastfeeding promotes skin-to-skin behavior also known as kangaroo care. Kangaroo care stabilizes your baby's heart and respiratory rates and regulates his or her blood sugar and body temperature. Skin-to-skin also improves oxygen saturation rates and conserves baby's calories. For women who are having trouble breastfeeding, many mothers find that latching their babies to the breast is easier after being held in kangaroo care. It can also calm a fussy baby.

Breastfeeding causes important immunological changes in your growing baby. When your body was sick and fought off illness, you built up a natural resistance to the disease. Those natural resistance cells are passed into your breast milk to build up your baby's immunity. Each teaspoon has three million antimicrobial cells in it! This means even a very small amount of breast milk each day is beneficial. Though older children breastfeed less, they receive a more concentrated dose of immune factors in breast milk.

Lactation protects against many diseases and conditions in the infant. This includes bacterial ear, respiratory tract, and urinary tract infections, as well as necrotizing enterocolitis and diarrhea. Breastfed babies grow up to receive a number of long-term benefits. They are less likely to develop childhood obesity, high blood pressure, and Type II Diabetes Mellitus. They receive a higher score on their Intelligent Quotient (IQ) tests. Breastfeeding for at least six months have lowered their risk for certain childhood cancers like neuroblastoma, leukemia, and Hodgkin's disease. Research shows that breast milk contains high levels of specific cancer-fighting cells called TNF-related apoptosis-inducing ligand (TRAIL).

Breastfeeding decreases a mother's risk for many diseases and condition, as well! This includes a decreased risk of postpartum hemorrhage and bleeding due to rapid uterine shrinking. Breastfeeding is also increased child spacing and decreased menstrual blood loss because increased prolactin delays the return of ovulation and menstruation. Moms who lactate enjoy a quicker return to pre-pregnancy weight and a decreased risk of breast and ovarian cancers.

Babies experience positive psychological effects of breastfeeding. Your baby moves from hearing the heartbeat in your snug, warm womb to the cold and bright light that overwhelms them. While breastfeeding, your baby gazes into your eyes and your presence reassures the baby. Breastfeeding promotes an emotional bond from both the physical closeness and the effects of the oxytocin.

Both international and national professional organizations recommend exclusive breastfeeding. The World Health Organization (WHO) defines breastfeeding as the "normal way of providing young infants with the nutrients they need for healthy growth and development".

The WHO believes that colostrum is the ideal baby food and babies should be breastfed within one hour of birth. Exclusive breastfeeding is recommended until 6 months of age. Continued breastfeeding with complementary baby foods is recommended until age two-years-old and beyond.

The American Academy Pediatrics (AAP) states that human milk is the superior form of infant feeding and recommends that exclusive breastfeeding should be used as the reference point that all other feeding methods should be measured against. The AAP also states that there are meaningful benefits to breastfed babies in terms of growth, developmental, and health, especially in the premature infant.

Chapter 17

Contraindication to Breastfeeding

There are conditions that the general public incorrectly believe are incompatible with breastfeeding. Contrary to popular belief, the following are not contraindicated. Mothers with hepatitis, including Hepatitis B surface antigen-positive, Hepatitis C virus antibody, and Hepatitis C virus RNA positive blood can all breastfeed. In mothers who are seropositive with cytomegalovirus (CMV), the benefits of breastfeeding outweigh the risks of transmission.

Some women may have detectable levels of chemical pollutants in their breast milk, but there are no laboratory guidelines to detect abnormal levels. Breast milk is not routinely tested for environmental contaminants. Mothers who have been exposed to low-level environmental chemical agents (like phthalates) should breastfeed because the benefits outweigh the risks.

Moms who are tobacco smokers can breastfeed. However, any smoking mother, regardless of feeding method, should make every effort to quit smoking. Mothers who smoke should not smoke in the house or around the baby and wash their hands, face, and clothes prior to picking up a baby.

Breastfeeding moms can drink alcohol in moderation. According to the AAP, alcohol is a medication that is usually compatible with breastfeeding, but excessive or regular drinking should be avoided. Alcohol is rapidly absorbed and cleared from milk. However, it can alter the taste of milk and inhibit milk production temporarily. Mothers should wait about two to three hours after drinking one alcoholic beverage before breastfeeding. If you drink enough alcohol to feel intoxicated, wait even longer before nursing the baby. Pumping will not remove alcohol from the milk, but if you are uncomfortable while waiting to breastfeed, you can pump until comfort.

Some mothers with fevers are worried that they should not breastfeed. Fevers can be caused by infections or mastitis (a breast infection). If you have caught a contagious infection, your baby is already at risk for transmission. They will benefit from the antibodies in your breast milk to help protect against the infection that you are carrying. If it is a breast infection, your baby nursing may help to clear the infection.

Finally, babies with jaundice can breastfeed. This condition is also known as hyperbilirubinemia. It is important to listen to your pediatrician as they may recommend specific feeding techniques or formula in addition to your breast milk.

True contraindications to breastfeeding are infants with classic galactosemia (known as Galactose 1-phosphate uridyltransferase deficiency) because they are unable to digest breast milk. American mothers who are infected with human immunodeficiency virus (HIV) should not breastfeed due to the risk of HIV transmission to the infant. Finally, certain medications are contraindicated in breastfeeding. Unfortunately, many healthcare providers are not educated in safe medications for lactation and err on the side of caution. Dr. Hale's Infant Risk website and hotline provide an excellent resource to assure that the medications you are taking are safe for breastfeeding.

You may not breastfeed due to choice, medical contraindication, or inability to produce enough supply. That is not something that should be cause for guilt or conflict. It is important to support one another's choices. Most parents are doing what is best for their babies and families. There are other healthy options to feed your baby.

Chapter 18

Exclusive Pumping

There are many situations where a mom may not nurse her baby but feel strongly about her baby getting her breast milk. A mother who has a baby who is premature, who cannot or will not latch, or who prefers not to have a baby at their breast may choose to exclusively pump her breasts. Exclusively pumping, known as "EPing" in some communities, is an exceptional way to provide nourishment to your babe.

Unfortunately, it does not always receive the support and acknowledgment that it deserves. Moms who exclusively pump have no need for "mom guilt". Typically, it is the most time consuming of the infant feeding options. Mom who EP are dedicated to feeding baby their breast milk.

Many people, including health care providers, are not well versed in the option. They may attempt to discourage mothers or offer infant formula as a viable option. Mothers going this route need support to continue pumping.

Moms who choose to exclusively pump may feel isolated, excluded from both breastfeeding and formula feeding mothers. They may feel defensive in their explanation about what substance is in their bottle or frustrated by health care providers and others who ask "breast or bottle"?

While feeding baby at the breast has unique benefits, breast milk itself is irreplaceable. If the choice is between breast milk and formula, one should always opt for breast milk, if able.

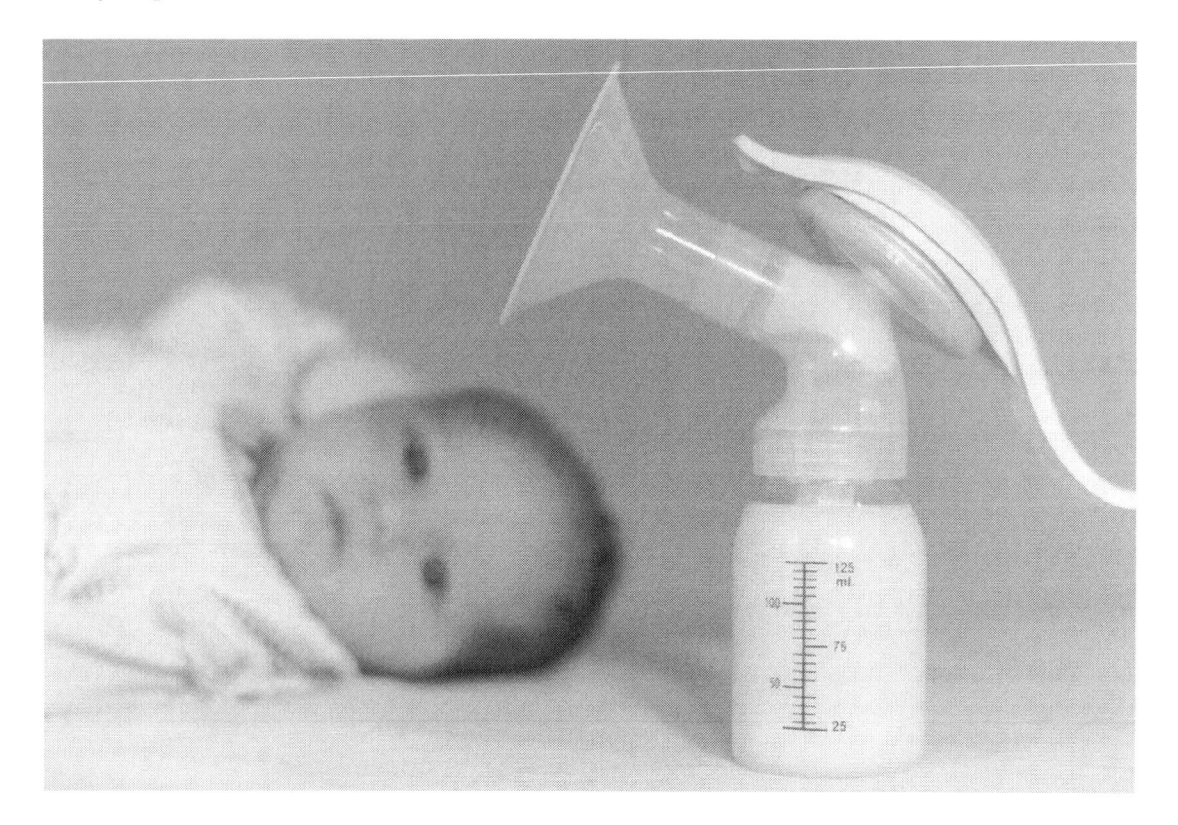

Moms who exclusively pump need a double electric pump. On average, a healthy infant breastfeeds 8 to 12 times per day. Moms who exclusively pump should strive to initially pump at the same frequency. You should pump every two hours, never allowing more than three hours between sessions. The more often that you empty your breasts, the more milk the mother will make.

Women should aim to pump 15 to 20 minutes per session, or about five minutes beyond the time the milk stops flowing to see if they can trigger a second letdown of milk. Prolactin is highest between one and five in the morning, so schedule one pump during that time period.

Another consideration while pumping is to set the strength of the suction to a comfortable level. If the suction is too strong, it can negatively affect your breast milk flow and cause injury to your nipple. A breastfed baby will typically drink about 19 to 30 ounces per day. Ideally, your breasts will create the same amount that your baby consumes.

Babies should be fed "on demand". This means you should feed your baby when they show hunger cues, but not on a rigid schedule. You should use slow flow nipples to simulate nursing from the breast. Spend time with your baby during the feeding session, aiming for a feed lasting 15 to 20 minutes.

All breastfeeding moms should focus on being well hydrated. You should aim to drink enough so you have clear yellow urine. It' important to avoid thirst, by the time you are thirsty you are often dehydrated. One should consume 8 to 16 ounces of water per nursing session. Stay nourished while eating healthy meals and frequent snacks. Traditional oatmeal from scratch (not in the package) is an excellent way to boost breast milk supply!

Congratulations!

The third character of the password required to unlock the Pregnancy Question & Answer booklet is letter n.

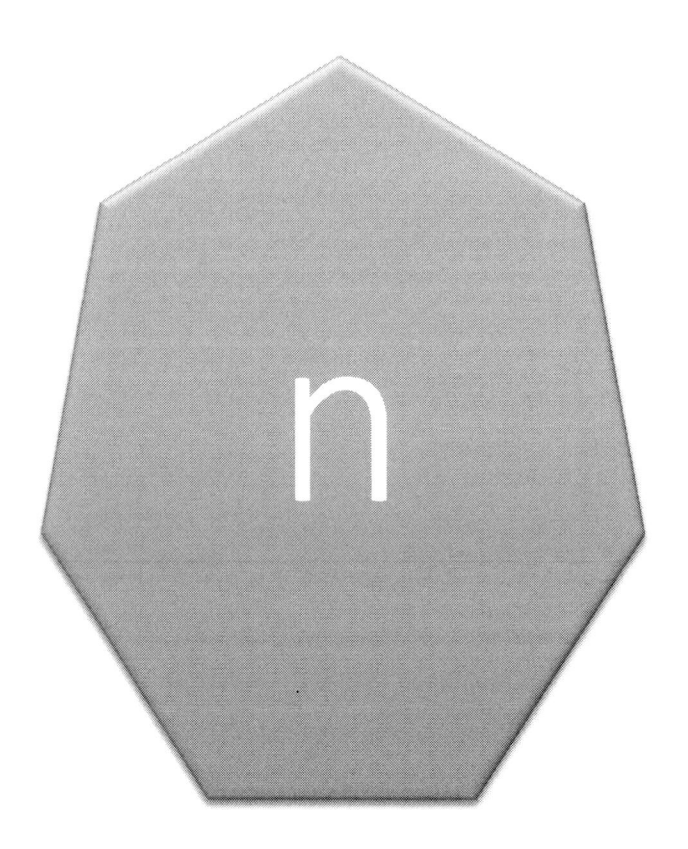

Chapter 19

Donor Breast Milk

Breast milk is the superior food for your new baby. If you choose not to breastfeed, need to supplement your nursing sessions, or are unable to make milk, donor milk may be a good option. It is typically available from a milk bank or hospital with a prescription. Your obstetrician, doctor, nurse-midwife, or pediatrician can write the prescription.

Donor milk is often an excellent choice for premature infants. Breast milk boosts a baby's immune system to fight illness, provides superior nutrition for growth and development, and can shorten their length of stay.

Unfortunately, breast milk is in short supply and donor banks are scarce in many locations. Donated breast milk is very safe. It comes from moms who are breastfeeding babies and make more milk than their baby can eat. Donors are tested for communicable illnesses that could pass through their breast milk, and each container of milk is tested for harmful bacteria.

Next, the donor milk is pasteurized to eliminate any risk of an infectious organism in the milk. Pasteurization destroys a small amount of the nutrients and antibodies in breast milk, but the milk retains a number of benefits. These benefits and nutrients cannot be replicated by infant formula.

Chapter 20

Bottle-feeding

Formula feeding is also a healthy option for babies and a viable alternative to breast milk. Infant formula has been scientifically tested and manufactured to have a healthy nutrient profile. If you prepare the infant formula correctly, it will minimize the risk of any infections to your baby. It is important to use manufacturer produced infant formula and not create your own. You should never substitute cow's milk for infant formula until your baby is one year old.

The benefits of bottle-feeding are that it is flexible and convenient. This means you can easily tailor a feeding schedule to your family. With infant formula, family members can easily feed the baby and you can schedule feedings at an ideal time because formula fed babies eat less frequently. Formula is a good option if a woman is opposed or unable to breast pump at work or feed in public.

It is important to choose one brand of infant formula and stick with it. If your baby appears to have gastrointestinal distress or fussiness on it, give it at least a week or two before you switch to a different brand. Babies truly need time for their bellies to adjust. Whatever you do, do not switch formula brands in less than one week.

There is premade formula or powdered formula that you reconstitute. There are a number of careful considerations for preparation of infant formula. The first step is hand washing. It is important to wash your hands with warm water and soap. You should wash your hands for the entire length of the song "Twinkle, Twinkle Little Star".

The powdered formula is usually prepared into a bottle for your baby with one scoop to two ounces of water. You can use any clean source of water to prepare the formula. You can use tap water, bottled water, nursery water, or faucet water to prepare formula.

Nursery water is fluoridated water made for younger babies. The concern with fluoridation is that it causes an increased risk for babies getting too much fluoride, which leads to dental fluorosis. In its mildest form, fluorosis usually appears as opaque white patches on enamel. In a more severe form, it leads to brown, mottled patches on the teeth that are permanent. Dentists advise that infant formula should be reconstituted with optimally fluoridated drinking water while being aware of the risks for your baby's enamel.

Powdered infant formula is not sterile. There is always the slight risk of it containing bacteria and being an infection risk for babies. It is imperative that formula is prepared correctly to reduce the risk of illness. Babies that are premature, low birth weight, and have compromised immune systems are more at risk for infection. Water should be no cooler than 70 degrees Fahrenheit.

It is important to make sure you are using one level scoop into premeasured two ounces of water. If you get the ratio incorrect, it could cause your infant to not get the proper nutrition.

Formula feeding is widely practiced in the United States. The goal is for six months of exclusive breastfeeding in the United States, but most women have supplemented their babies with formula by six months. Some literature connects the spike in formula feeding to contribute to the development of population disease, including allergic reactions, Type II Diabetes Mellitus, and childhood obesity.

There is no reason to be ashamed if you are unable or unwilling to breastfeed. There is a lot of pressure to breastfeed. Women who have just given birth are already at risk for postpartum depression and anxiety. Feeling like a failure is not helpful to one's mind.

There is so much guilt and worry about being a mother. While breast milk is created by nature for infants, modern infant formula is a perfectly acceptable alternative. It has been scientifically tested and modified to be a viable choice. Mothers should not feel any less if they opt to stop breastfeeding because they are becoming depressed or overwhelmed. A happy mommy means a happy baby.

Breastfeeding Positions

Breastfeeding is a skill that both mom and baby must learn. It requires extensive education and practice to become a skilled breastfeeding mother. Fortunately, there are a number of options when it comes to breastfeeding holds and positions. These positions involve football hold, cradle and cross cradle, side-lying, and laid back breastfeeding.

Each position has specific benefits and detriments. It can be awkward at first to find the best position for you and your baby to breastfeed in. If you experiment with several positions, eventually you will find the hold that works best for the two of you.

a) Football Hold

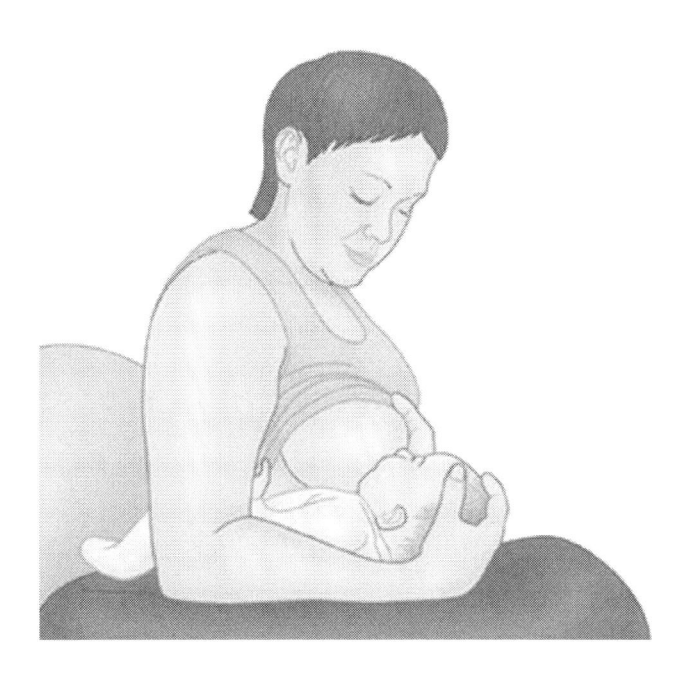

The football hold is the ideal position for moms who have a scar from their cesarean section surgical birth. In this hold, you sit up straight and place your baby beside you with your elbow bent. Your baby's toes should be pointed towards your back with baby curled around your side. You must support your baby's head and face her towards your breast with your baby's back on your forearm.

For cesarean section mamas, this position is typically the most comfortable seated position and does not put pressure on the scar on the abdomen. This breastfeeding position is easily done with nursing pillows, especially if you rotate the pillow to support your baby's head and body.

Football hold makes it easy to steady your baby's head to enable a wide-open latch as you bring the baby to your breast. In this position, babies often latch better and seem cozier as they are tightly wrapped around their mom. The football hold is compatible with smaller babies. It is ideal for moms with larger breasts who are struggling in other positions.

There are several drawbacks for moms who use football hold. These include the fact that a sleepy baby might fall asleep due to feeling too cozy. Depending on baby's size and mom's breast size, football hold may be tricky in public. Finally, it is difficult to do football hold with older babies and young children. Most mothers find themselves shifting away from this position as their baby grows.

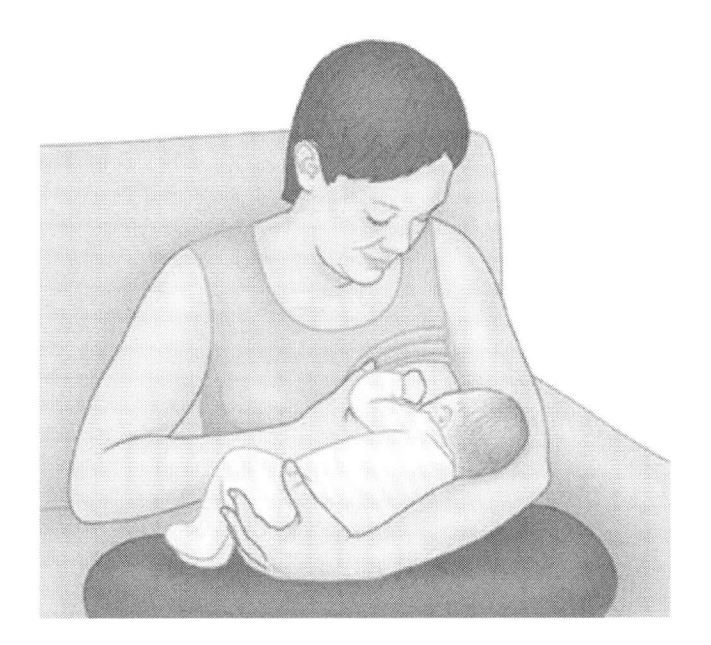

b) Cradle Hold

Cradle hold is an early breastfeeding position that enables you to support your baby's head in the crook of your arm. This is one of the first breastfeeding holds that many moms attempt. The cradle hold means that the baby's head in the crook of your arm on the same side as the breast you are feeding on. If you are nursing on the right breast, the baby's head is in the crook of the right arm.

To perform this breastfeeding hold, sit up straight. Start by cradling your baby in your right arm with your baby's head resting comfortably on your elbow. Turn the baby's face to your breast and place the baby tummy to tummy. Bring the baby to your breast to nurse, do not bring your breast to the baby! You can use a pillow on your lap to support the baby and prevent yourself from hunching over. This is similar to the next position, the cross-cradle hold.

c) Cross-Cradle Hold

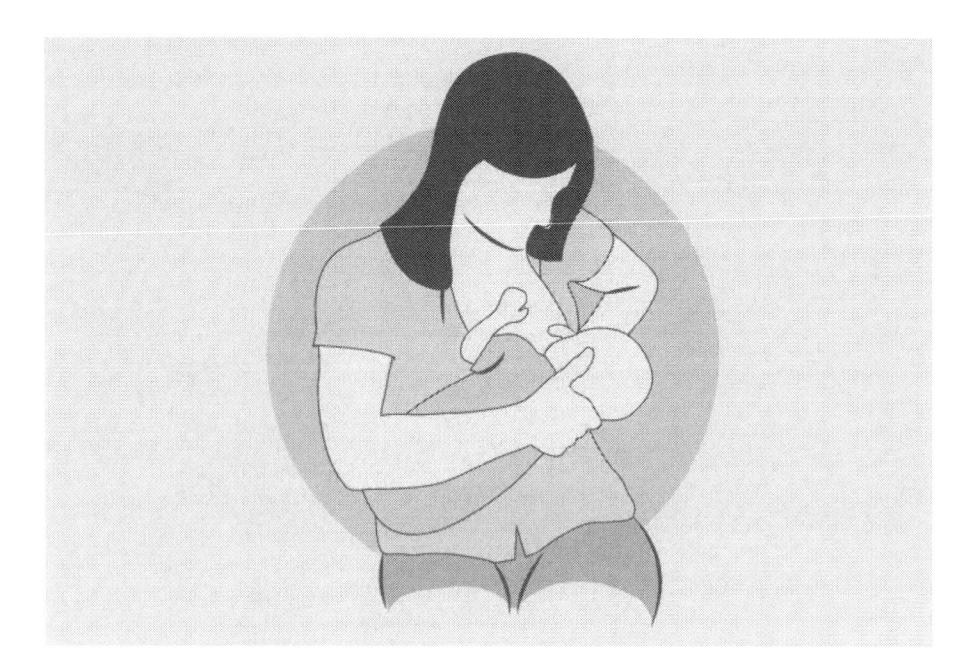

Cross-cradle hold is also known as crossover hold and is ideal for early breastfeeding. It is the exact opposite of cradle hold. Sit up straight in a comfortable chair and bring the baby across your body. It is important to always maintain contact between the baby's tummy and yours. Hold your baby in the crook of the arm opposite from the breast that you are feeding your baby from. If you are nursing on your left breast, hold your baby in your right arm. If you are nursing on your right breast, hold your baby in your left arm.

With the other hand, make your fingers into a U shape and support directly underneath the breast you are feeding your baby on. Guide the baby's mouth to your breast. Do not bend over, lean forward, or pull your breast to the baby's mouth. Cradle the baby close to your chest. Support the baby's skull just below the curve towards the neck as to not disturb your baby during the feed.

If the crossover hold is used improperly, it can cause the baby to nurse poorly and break their latch. Make sure to sit up straight and bring the baby to you. A concern for this hold is back pain from poor posture. Your shoulder and arm may begin to ache. Reposition, using pillows or shifting your hold. If you do not reposition and your arm is in pain, it may cause the nipple to start to slide to the front of the baby's mouth. The other concern is that the wrist supporting the baby's head is at risk for injury. This wrist pain is a concern with the aforementioned cradle hold, as well. Try to use the ideal position to promote ideal posture and decrease back pain.

d) Laid Back Breastfeeding

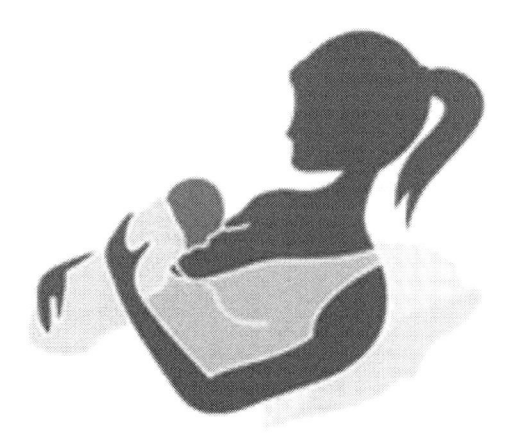

This type of breastfeeding is also known as biological nurturing. Mom should recline in an armchair, sofa, or on the bed propped up by pillows. It is important for mom to choose the place where she feels the most comfortable.

Baby is placed on mom's tummy to baby's tummy. The baby can approach the nipple from any of the 360 degrees surrounding the breast and still get a good latch. This includes baby lying vertically below mother's breast, diagonally below the breasts, across the breasts, at her side, or even over the shoulder.

Laid-back breastfeeding is less work for moms and allows young babies to take the breast deeply. This is the perfect position for new moms to relax and put their feet up or catch a nap while they nurse. (Note: If you are going to nap, make sure that you are with a trusted family member to ensure that your baby is in a safe position.) It is helpful to have a support person to assist with positioning the baby at the breast at first.

In the beginning, gravity helps rather than hinders your baby's feeding reflexes. This position promotes cuddling, relaxation, and breastfeeding. Often mom and baby are able to find the best position by trial and error. The best part about this breastfeeding hold is that there is a variety of options in which babies can approach the breast

This increases opportunities for that valuable skin-to-skin time with your new baby. It also allows babies to snuggle with mom on their tummies. This position allows baby to direct the breastfeeding session and is ideal for moms with oversupply or forceful letdown, as gravity slows down the flow of milk for your baby. Laid-back breastfeeding can be used for babies and toddlers of all ages and sizes. Since you are not hunched over your baby in an awkward seated position, laid-back breastfeeding reduces back pain. The only drawback for this breastfeeding hold is that it is hard to perform laidback breastfeeding in public while you are outside of the house.

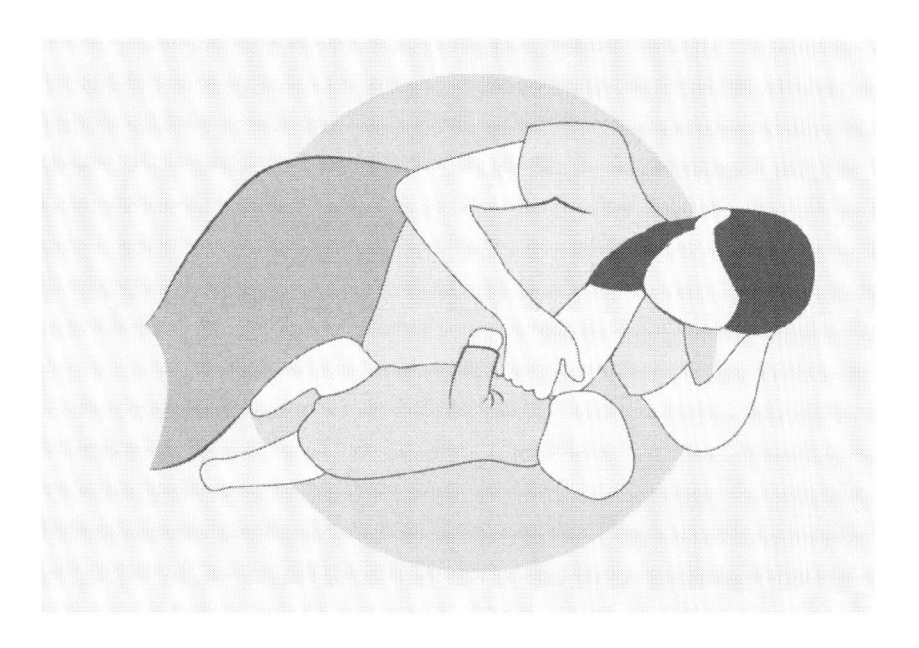

e) Side-lying

Side-lying hold is a position where you are able to lie on your side and you're your baby toward your breast. This is a position that provides an intimate relationship with your newborn. Make sure baby is snuggled close to you and support the baby with one hand. Grab your breast with the other hand and put your nipple to the baby's lips. After the baby latches, use that arm to support your own head.

This breastfeeding position is good for moms with painful lacerations or swollen bottoms after birth. It allows mothers to avoid sitting for long periods of time. It is also the best position to take a nap while you are breastfeeding. You can also do side-lying breastfeeding with a child of any age. The drawback is that it is difficult to do in public.

There are many breastfeeding holds that have different advantages and weaknesses. It is so important to find the best breastfeeding positions that work for you and your baby. Moms who bottle-feed are not told how to hold their baby. They learn based on trial and error. You can find the best position by attempting the holds and seeing what works. It is best to have plenty of information and support concerning breastfeeding.

If you are having trouble breastfeeding, it is imperative that you get lactation support as soon as possible. There are private postpartum doulas that can provide you and your baby with TLC. There is the La Leche League, which has local meetings. The meeting times vary from several times per week to once a month. You can also check your local hospital to see if they have a breastfeeding support group.

If your need for breastfeeding help is immediate or specific, you should look into a breastfeeding counselor or lactation consultant. A breastfeeding expert can provide personalized assistance and knowledge. A breastfeeding counselor is a support person who is trained in breastfeeding encouragement and can troubleshoot initial breastfeeding problems. An International Board Certified Lactation Consultant (IBCLC) is a healthcare professional, often a Registered Nurse, specializing in the more advanced management of lactation issues. These lactation consultants can work at hospitals, doctor offices, clinics, and private practice.

Some health insurance companies will completely cover lactation services. Call your health insurance provider for local lactation consultants and you're your insurance coverage benefits allow. Lactating moms are likely to be successful at breastfeeding if armed with a wealth of information and the support of their family, health care providers, and society.

Chapter 21

Breastfeeding Diet

Creating milk for your infant is intense work for your body. It is important to provide enough hydration and nourishment to make adequate milk for your baby. While you can eat and drink what you like while breastfeeding, you should aim to eat as well as possible. You should always eat processed foods in moderation and be cautious about consuming an abundance of sweets. Even if you cannot eat properly, your baby will always get the best possible nutrition from your body. However, your body may suffer from your baby getting all of the good nutrients. If you eat well, you both will benefit from suitable nutrition.

Lactation increases your caloric energy needs by about 500 calories per day. These calories should come from a healthy and varied diet. Breastfeeding leads to an increased need for most macronutrients, minerals, and vitamins. Primarily focus on a balanced diet involving fruits, vegetables, lean meats, dairy, healthy fats from sources like nuts, avocado, almonds, and peanut butter. It is important to hydrate well with fluids like water and milk.

Snacks for the Breastfeeding Mother

2 Hard boiled eggs + a glass of chocolate milk	Whole grain crackers with nut butter + a glass of milk
Cottage cheese + fresh fruit and veggie toppings	Hummus + fresh veggies or whole grain crackers
Greek yogurt + fresh fruit	Nut Butter + celery

| Nut butter + apples or bananas | Water infused with lemon, strawberry, or kiwi |

Breastfeeding moms do not have to specifically avoid any food. However, if you are noticing that your baby is fussy or gassy, some moms opt to try to eliminate particular foods from their diet. In reality, any food could be the culprit. However, there are some foods that are more likely to cause gastrointestinal distress. These foods include:

- spices (cinnamon, garlic, curry, chili pepper)
- citrus fruits or juice (oranges, lemons, limes, and grapefruit)
- some fruits (strawberries, kiwifruit, pineapple, cherry, prunes)
- the "gassy" veggies (onion, cabbage, garlic, cauliflower, broccoli, cucumbers, and peppers)

Supplementation

Vitamin D is necessary for you and your baby's body to absorb calcium and foster bone growth. A deficiency in Vitamin D puts children at risk for Ricketts and adults at risk for osteomalacia (misshapen bones). Having low vitamin D also causes fatigue, bone pain, difficulty thinking, and muscle weakness. It is very important that both you and your baby receive adequate Vitamin D supplementation.

Breastfeeding moms should supplement their baby with 400 units of Vitamin D drops. Breastfeeding moms are also in need of supplementation for themselves.

New research shows that mom taking 6400 units of Vitamin D per day is a safe and effective alternative to baby taking drops.

Breastfeeding Tips

While breastfeeding is a normal and natural act, many women find it harder than they originally thought it would be. Being prepared is the best way to ensure that you are able to breastfeed. The frequently asked questions in the following section will help prepare you to breastfeed your baby.

Chapter 22

Frequently Asked Questions

1. How do I know my breastfed infant is getting enough milk?

You will be able to determine that your infant is drinking enough breast milk by seeing how many wet and dirty diapers that your baby is having. Your baby will have one dirty diaper for each day of life until day four when they should have three to four stools per day. Babies may also stool every time they nurse or more often. Baby's stool should be seedy, soft or runny after your milk comes in.

After birth, your baby should have one wet diaper for each day of life. Once mom's milk comes in, your baby should have six wet diapers every 24 hours. Health care providers will also evaluate your baby's weight gain to ensure they are getting enough breast milk (see next answer).

2. What is the average breastfed baby weight gain?

A normal infant will lose up to 7% of their birth weight in the first few days. Your pediatrician may become concerned if your baby loses more than 10%. After your breast milk comes in, the average breastfed baby will gain about six ounces per week. Baby should have a weight check at the end of the first week. If the baby is having trouble gaining weight, follow up with a lactation consultant and pediatrician.

3. How do you know if you have low milk supply?

Unfortunately, many mother's concerns that they have an insufficient milk supply will cause them to unnecessarily supplement with formula. Supplementation is a slippery slope to actually causing a supply issue. These misperceptions surrounding milk supply issues cause mothers to stop breastfeeding prior to twelve months. With generations of bottle-feeding mothers before us, the knowledge of how a normal, breastfed infant behaves has been lost.

The breast pump is not a good indicator of your milk supply. Many mothers think that their milk supply is low and it is actually not. If your baby is gaining weight and having enough wet and dirty diapers on breast milk alone, then you do not have a problem with milk supply.

4. What are reasons for low milk supply?

Breast milk supply is based on supply and demand. You must remove more milk from the breast to encourage the development of more breast milk. It is important to do it more frequently. If your baby is not removing enough milk effectively from your breast, then your supply will decrease.

The following are some of the reasons your baby may not be removing milk effectively:

- Your baby's latch or positioning is not ideal

- A baby who is difficult to wake up

- Nipple shields

- Anatomical problems in baby (cleft palate or lip, lip tie, tongue tie)

- Stopping nursing before baby is done actively nursing

- Breastfeeding less than every 2-3 hours

- Using a pacifier and bottle

- Supplementing with formula, solids, or water.

- Maternal health issues, malnourishment, or dehydration.

5. How do you increase breast milk supply?

If baby has a poor latch or is often sleepy, express milk after or between feedings to maintain a milk supply. You can either hand express or use a breast pump.

- Begin pumping in order to remove milk from the breasts to trigger an increase in supply. Keep pumping about five minutes after the last drops fall. However, even a short pumping session is helpful if you are limited on time.

- Switch sides three or more times per feeding particularly every you're your baby's suckling slows down or she falls asleep. Use each side twice per feeding.

- Nurse frequently (every 90 minutes to two hours) and continue through the entire time the baby is actively nursing.

- Try power pumping. Pick one hour and pump for 20 minutes, rest 10 minutes, pump another 10 minutes, rest 10 minutes, pump 10 minutes.

- Galactagogues are supplements that increase breast milk supply. They may be like a Band-Aid to the underlying problem. Some supplements to try are oatmeal, fenugreek, alfalfa, fennel, and blessed thistle.

6. Should I supplement with infant formula?

If your baby is healthy, gaining weight, and having enough wet and dirty diapers, the answer is no. In general, the supplementation with infant formula is a slippery slope. The more that you supplement, the more it affects future breast milk supply.

In some cases, a pediatrician may recommend supplementation. The only time supplementation is medically indicated is when:

- Your baby has a significant weight loss of more than 10% in the newborn infant
- Babies with slow or no weight gain
- Serious illness or health issues in mom or baby
- Physical problems with mom or baby
- Breast refusal
- Separation of mother and baby (work or travel)
- critically dehydrated infants
- Adoption
- Very low birth weight

- Severe dysmaturity of the newborn with possible hypoglycemia
    - Syndrome associated with post-maturity and placental insufficiency
    - Babies have little subcutaneous fat, skin wrinkling, prominent nails, meconium staining of skin and placenta
- Infants with inherited metabolism syndrome
- mothers taking contraindicated medication with no safe alternative

7. Are special precautions needed for handling breast milk?

No, you do not need to adhere to specific guidelines to handle breast milk. Wash your hands with warm water and soap before pumping and handling breast milk. You should also start with clean bottles or new bags and pump parts. Label and date the bottle or bag of breast milk, always using the oldest breast milk bag first. It is important to clean your pump parts after each pumping session with hot water and detergent. Rinse them thoroughly with hot water. Dry them.

Breast milk can be stored in the general home or work refrigerator. Some women choose to place it in an insulated lunch bag with ice packs and keep it on their desk. Some will let it sit at their desk for a limited amount of time. You can add newly pumped breast milk to the milk that is already in the refrigerator, but you must cool it first.

Breast Milk Storage Guidelines

Room Temperature	Six hours
Insulated bag with ice packs	24 hours
Refrigerator (back of fridge)	5 days
Home Freezer Compartment	14 days
Home Freezer	6 months

5. Why do my nipples hurt?

In the beginning, it is normal to have some pain and tenderness for the first few seconds when the baby latches. If the pain continues throughout the feeding, it may be the sign of a problem. Babies with tongue or lip-ties, a shallow latch, and thrush may cause nipple pain. It can also occur with breast pump trauma.

There are an unlucky few who may experience pain with breastfeeding through the entire breastfeeding relationship. If you have evaluated your baby's latch and ruled out any concerns, your nipples may be sensitive to suction.

6. What is cluster feeding?

Cluster feeding is when your baby nurses between frequent to near constantly for hours at a time. This breastfeeding usually occurs in the evenings and may coincide with your baby behaving in a fussy manner. These behaviors usually go hand in hand with growth spurts, characterized by more often nursing for several days. It may seem exhausting and frustrating. However, they pass within a few days. The purpose of cluster feeding is to increase your milk supply.

7. How do I awaken my sleeping baby to feed him?

In order to wake your baby up before a feed, try changing your baby's diaper. It will often wake up your infant. You can also clap your baby's hands together or gently bicycle the baby's legs. Rub the soles of your baby's feet or gently massage your baby's scalp. You can also do "baby sit-ups", where you support the baby's head and lift the head and shoulders while the rest of the body lies down, are a gentle way to wake your baby. If the baby falls asleep when you are breastfeeding, you can switch the baby to the other breast.

8. Is it okay to nurse in public? Should I nurse in front of my family?

Nursing in public is an absolutely wonderful choice that is entirely up to you and your comfort level. The law in nearly all states protects it and public nursing is becoming more widespread. It is important to have the flexibility to breastfeed when you are out and about.

If you want to be a breastfeeding advocate, nurse in the same room as family and friends. You may nurse covered or uncovered. However, the more that people are exposed to breastfeeding, the more normal they will begin to see it.

9. Do I really have to pump every 2 to 3 hours if I am exclusively pumping?

Yes, you absolutely do in the beginning. The same goes for nursing every 2 to 3 hours initially if you are exclusively breastfeeding. It all comes back to supply and demand. The more you ask of your breasts, the more they will give! It is important to encourage more milk production by breastfeeding or pumping your breasts as much as possible.

10. What can I put on my sore nipples?

Honestly, the best thing to put on your sore nipples is breast milk. Squeeze a bit out, leave it on the nipples, and leave them open to air. However, lanolin cream and is also an option for pain. If you do not have nipple cream at home, try organic coconut oil or olive oil. The best part about these ointments is that you do not have to worry about wiping the lanolin, oil, or breast milk off in between breastfeeding sessions. Leave them on the breast open to air and nurse your baby.

11. What do I do if my baby skips a feed?

First of all, the most important part is to try to prevent your baby from missing a feed. You should try to do everything possible to get your baby to nurse. Try the aforementioned tips to wake a sleepy baby. If you are still unable to get your baby to breastfeed, make sure to pump after the feeding to make sure your supply keeps up. Pump at least 15 to 25 minutes for each breastfeeding session.

12. What if breastfeeding does not work out for us?

Being a mom is hard work. Breastfeeding is stressful and complicated. While it is often worth it in the end, sometimes the stress is not worth it. Sometimes you are unable to make enough breast milk to support your baby. If breastfeeding does not work out, it is okay. You are the perfect mother for your baby. Your baby will still be healthy and your sanity is the most important factor. If you are a happy, sane mother, your baby will benefit.

13. When should a baby start solid foods?

A baby should not start solid foods until at least six months. Until then, a baby should be exclusively breastfed or given infant formula. You can start complementary solid foods at six months, but breastfeeding (or formula feeding) should continue until at least one year. Moms who wish to breastfeed longer because it is mutually beneficial are absolutely appropriate.

14. How long should a mother breastfeed?

The American Academy of Pediatrics (AAP) recommends a minimum of breastfeeding through one year of age. The World Health Organization recommends through at least two years old. You should breastfeed as long as you can. It should be comfortable and beneficial for both you and your baby.

15. Will my baby breastfeed forever?

It may seem that you will breastfeed forever. You will not breastfeed until college and you will absolutely sleep again. You can rest assured that your baby will eventually wean as your baby sees fit. It's also okay if you don't want to leave it to baby's timing. Babies typically wean any time after their first birthday through four years old.

16. Should I give formula before bed to help my baby sleep through the night?

You should not give infant formula to help your baby sleep through the night. It will not help! The thought is that formula is broken down less easily than breast milk and that babies will sleep longer when they have it their stomach. The truth is that breastfed babies may wake up because they long for the comfort of breastfeeding. The need for comfort from mom will not be dissuaded by formula feeding. If your infant is successfully nursing, a bottle of formula at night will not help your baby sleep better. However, it may negatively affect your supply and set you up for breastfeeding issues down the road.

17. What is a tongue-tie or lip-tie?

Everyone has a labial (lip) and lingual (tongue) frenulum, which is a tissue connection to your mouth. The difference between a normal frenulum and a tongue and lip-tie are how the tie functions and if it interferes with feeding. A tongue and lip tie involves a tight frenulum. This tight band of tissue prevents a proper latch. There are several ways to assess whether a baby has a tongue-tie or lip-tie. These include:

- Can you see or feel a tight lip or tongue frenulum?

- Does your baby have a high or narrow roof of his or her mouth?

- Does your baby's tongue rise less than halfway to the roof of the mouth while crying?

- Do the sides of your baby's tongue lift, but not the center of the tongue?

- Does the tip of the tongue look heart-shaped?

You can see a tongue or lip-tie best when the infant is crying. It is important to assess the mouth at that time.

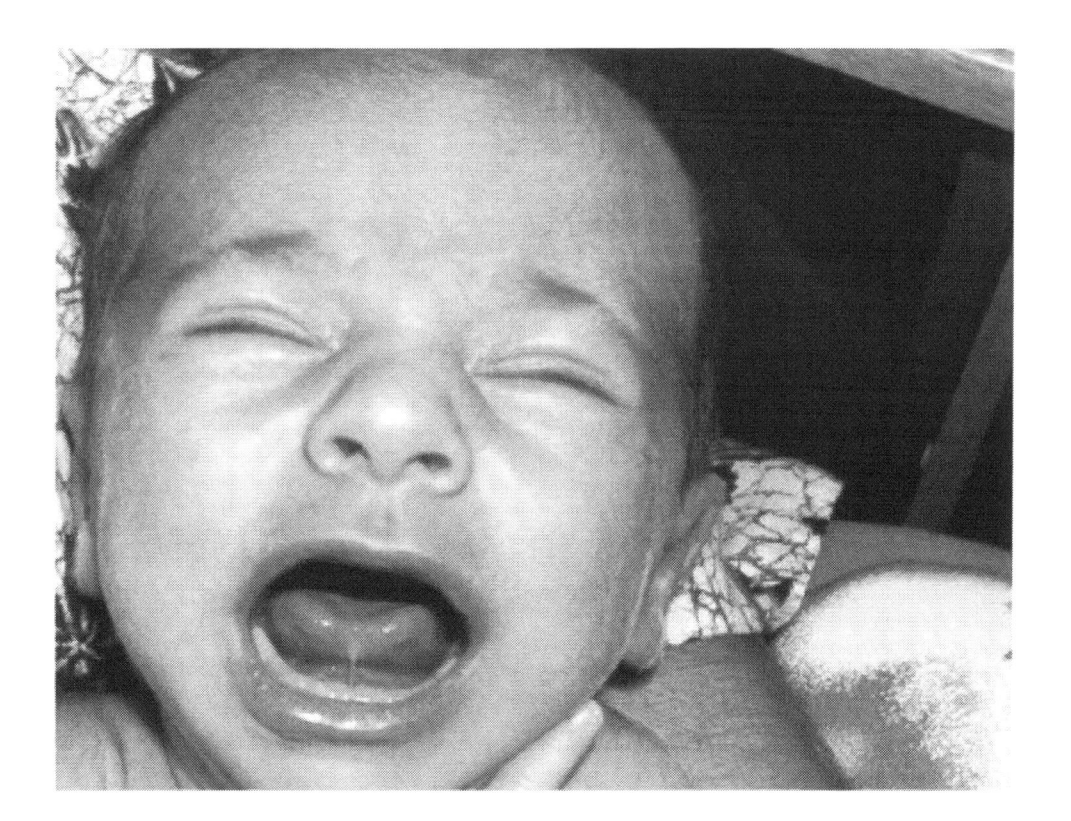

18. What are the drawbacks of a tongue-tie or lip-tie?

There are a number of drawbacks for tongue-tie and lip-tie. These can be common causes of breastfeeding issues for mothers, like breast pain, engorgement, uneven breast milk transfer, and nipple pain. It can cause mom to have nipple bruising, creasing, or erosions. It can cause a white stripe on the nipple, vasospasm, or thrush. It also plugged ducts, mastitis, and early weaning. It also can cause your baby to have issues like slow weight gain, and low milk supply.

Babies may have a poor latch, make a clicking sound while nursing, a painful or strong suck, poor transfer of milk, and decreased swallowing after let-down. These babies have symptoms of colic, reflux, fussiness, and irritability. Babies with a tongue or lip-tie cough, choke, gulp, spill milk during feeds, and experiencing jaw quivering during her feeds. They become sleepy during feeds, bite on the nipple, and slide off the breasts

19. Can a tongue-tie or lip-tie be fixed?

Yes, a tongue-tie or lip-tie absolutely can be fixed in a quick outpatient procedure. The surgery is performed by surgical instruments or laser and called a frenotomy. Many parents report immediate improvement in breastfeeding after the revision of the tie. The major barricade to fixing a tongue or lip-tie is that many physicians do not properly assess or diagnose a tongue or lip-tie. Some lactation consultants are skilled at recognizing these, while others are not.

If you believe your child has a tongue or lip-tie, it is important to be diligent about getting a second opinion.

Chapter 23

Myths and Misperceptions

1. Breast augmentation or reduction surgery prevents your ability to breastfeed.

A breast augmentation or reduction surgery does not disqualify you from breastfeeding. Many women are able to breastfeed successfully after breast and nipple surgery. Depending on the type of surgery that was performed, you should be able to produce some amount of breast milk. Even a small amount of breast milk has amazing biologic, immunologic, and maternal bonding qualities for your baby. While the surgery may impair your ability to breastfeed, most women do not know if they can nurse until they try. Breast reduction surgery appears to affect lactation ability the most.

2. Moms who smoke cannot breastfeed.

Moms who smoke can and absolutely should breastfeed, according to the American Academy of Pediatrics. While there is a lot of concerning data about second-hand smoke, it is actually beneficial for a baby who is at risk for tobacco exposure to be protected with breast milk. Likewise, any smoking mother should be instructed to quit smoking. If the parent is unwilling or unable to quit smoking, they should be educated about tobacco cessation to promote their baby's health. It is important to never smoke around the baby and do their best to wash off any second-hand smoke before holding the baby.

3. Breastfeeding mothers cannot consume alcohol.

Breastfeeding mothers who consume alcohol in moderation can continue to breastfeed. The recommendation is to breastfeed immediately prior to drinking an alcoholic beverage and waiting two to three hours before nursing. If you are intoxicated, you should have someone else watch your infant. Breastfeeding while consuming alcohol should be questioned if you binge drink.

If you have small breasts, it significantly affects your ability to make milk.
The amount of milk a mother can make has nothing to do with breast size. Women with very small breasts are able to breastfeed successfully.

4. You have to consume a special diet for breastfeeding.

It is important to eat healthfully since you are nourishing two people. However, even with an imperfect diet, your body will make the perfect food for your baby. Your body may be left to suffer if you eat poorly. The most important consideration is to stay hydrated and to eat enough food to be well nourished.
If baby is fussy two to twelve hours after you eat specific foods, you may consider cutting them out.

5. I have to stop breastfeeding because my baby has a milk allergy.

If your baby is having a dairy allergy, he or she is not allergic to the breast milk itself, but allergic to cows milk protein in the breast milk. Cutting out cow's milk from your diet will help your allergic baby. However, it can take several days to notice an improvement in your baby's symptoms. You do not need to stop breastfeeding because of an allergy. Allergen friendly formula is extremely expensive. If you believe that your baby has a dairy allergy, it is best to see if you can eliminate dairy from your diet for a full week before switching to formula.

6. Every baby's feeding schedule is the same and should be two to three hours apart.

In a textbook, every breastfeeding mom should breastfeed every two to three hours. This minimum time between feeds is the absolute recommendation. However, the true recommendation is 8 to 12 times per day initially. This can be done at any spacing.

Some babies may want to feed every hour for four hours. Some babies may have a period of time where they go four hours without breastfeeding, but the rest of the feeds are closer together. Listen to your babies hunger cues to determine the best schedule for you and your baby.

Feeding a baby "on demand" is often the best solution. This means that you will feed the baby when showing hunger cues. Hunger cues include sucking a fist, putting fingers in his or her mouth, and smacking the baby's lips.

7. Breastfed babies should never use a pacifier.

Early on, pacifier use should be avoided. However, studies have been done on pacifiers and their effect on breastfeeding. In some cases, pacifier use appears to have almost no effect on breastfeeding. The lack of influence from pacifier use is only seen when mom has a strong desire to breastfeed and the pacifier has been introduced after breastfeeding has been well established and is going very well

8. Exclusively breastfed babies will not sleep through the night.

Some breastfed babies sleep through the night and some do not. In fact, if your baby is waking up to nurse at night and it is not a major problem for you, you do not have to try to change anything! While doctors, nurses, or family may tell you that night breastfeeding is not needed, nursing on cue will not hurt anyone. In fact, you are teaching your baby security, that you are there for her when she needs you. If it is a problem, listen to your health care providers and find a way to encourage your baby to sleep through the night.

9. If you are breastfeeding, you do not need birth control

If you want to avoid pregnancy, you should plan a backup method. If your baby is under six months old and you are breastfeeding exclusively, this is considered a form of birth control called the lactational amenorrhea method. This method is a temporary form of birth control that relies on the hormonal suppression of ovulation from exclusive breastfeeding. If you don't ovulate, you cannot get pregnant. It can be used from birth up to six months afterward.

With perfect use, the failure rate of lactational amenorrhea method is less than two percent. This method is only effective if you are not going longer than four hours without breastfeeding during the day or six hours at night. In order for this method to be successful, you must not have had a menstrual period, not be supplementing with formula or infant food, or having a baby who sleeps greater than four hours at a time during the day (or six hours during the night).

10. If you are breastfeeding, you cannot use birth control.

While experts recommend that you avoid combined oral contraceptive birth control pills while breastfeeding, most other forms of birth control are fine. You can still have a long acting method like an intrauterine device (IUDs) or a hormonal birth control implant in your arm. There are a variety of IUDs including ones with hormones that last between three to six years and a copper IUD with no hormones that lasts up to ten years. The implant in the arm is effective for three years.

There are shorter acting hormonal birth control options. These are also safe for breastfeeding. You can have the progestin injection known as Depo-Provera every three months. There is also the daily progesterone only pill that must be taken at the same time each day. This method is very tough for some with a new baby upending the schedule. There is also any barrier method like a diaphragm or condoms.

11. If you breastfeed, your breasts will sag.

If you have had a baby, your breasts have already changed in shape. Breastfeeding does not cause a long-term change in breast shape or elasticity, but pregnancy, genetics, and weight gain during pregnancy will. Some women's breasts return to their pre-breastfeeding shape or size. Your breasts may shrink or remain large.

12. Breastfeeding in public is shameful and should be avoided at all costs.

Breastfeeding is one of the most natural and nurturing acts that a mother can do with her baby. Our society has sexualized breasts, yet acts like breasts used to feed a child are appalling.

The good news is that breastfeeding in public is becoming increasingly prevalent. The more people who are exposed to it as a normal act, the more who will be informed. In fact, it is your legal right in most states. If your baby is hungry and you are comfortable, you should feed your baby with or without a nursing cover.

13. If you are sick you should stop breastfeeding.

If you are sick, you were most likely contagious several days ago. You most likely have already passed any disease to your baby. While your body is fighting against infectious invaders, your body will create antibodies to the infection. Your breast milk will pass the protective antibodies to your baby to keep your baby healthy.

Since it is already too late to avoid giving your baby the illness, is there anything that you can do? Wash your hands frequently, cover your cough or sneeze into your elbow, and breastfeed your baby as frequently as possible to keep him or her as healthy as possible.

14. Breastfeed past one-year-old is discouraged.

The World Health Organization recommends that you breastfeed your toddler until at least two years old or longer, if still mutually beneficial. Many women breastfeed for extended periods of time, including three to four years old. Breastfeeding duration is a decision that should be left to you and your child. If breastfeeding past two years old feels right for the two of you, then it is healthy, safe, and recommended.

15. Medications should be avoided with nursing.

Many medications pass into your breast milk, but most have no effect on your milk supply or on your baby. Most medications are safe with breastfeeding. However, there are some that should absolutely be avoided. Unfortunately, health care providers who do not frequently deal with lactating women do not always know what is safe. They may recommend that you stop breastfeeding or pump and dump to err on the side of caution.

There are a number of considerations to determine if a medication is safe for breastfeeding. This includes the amount of drug excreted into human milk, the extent that your baby will absorb the medication, and the risk of adverse effects from the medication to the infant.

There is an important resource for medications that are compatible with breastfeeding Dr. Hale's Infant Risk Center. The Infant Risk Center is available on the internet and by the hotline. The center has the most recent research regarding what medications are safe for breastfeeding your baby. If a medication is not safe for breastfeeding, they may be able to recommend a better alternative.

16. Sore nipples are completely normal.

Sore nipples are not normal. Tender nipples can happen in the beginning while your nipples are adjusting to breastfeeding. They may happen if your baby has a poor latch or your breasts have a blister or infection. Some women even continue to have a slight tenderness when they initiate breastfeeding even months after beginning. Most of these are outliers.

If you are having nipple pain, speak with a lactation consultant to ensure your baby has a good, open latch. Sore nipples are not a normal part of breastfeeding.

Chapter 24

Breastfeeding Accessories

Once you feel competent with breastfeeding, it is pretty clear-cut and hassle-free. One of the benefits of nursing is that it significantly cuts down on the amount of equipment you need to drag around. Initially, breastfeeding gear may make your feeding time more convenient and enjoyable. These are a few of the best items for breastfeeding mothers.

1. Breastfeeding pillow

A breastfeeding pillow will prevent you from poor posture while you breastfeed. Long breastfeeding sessions lead to hunching over your back causing stress on your shoulders and spine. Poor posture for twenty to thirty minutes for eight to twelve nursing sessions per day can negatively affect your back. A breastfeeding pillow raises your baby to the level of your breasts and provides support to minimize back pain and discomfort.

2. Breast pads

Breast pads are absorbent circles of material that go in your bra and absorb breast milk leakage. They will prevent any embarrassing leaks and wet spots. There are cloth pads that can be washed and disposable ones that can be thrown out. There is also something called milk savers that preserve extra milk that may leak out.

3. Milk-saver

A milk-saver goes in your bra on the non-nursing side while you breastfeed or pump your breasts. It collects any milk that leaks during letdown. Transfer the collected milk to your fridge or freezer to feed your baby later. It allows you to effortlessly store extra breast milk with each feeding. For mothers who are returning to work, this is an excellent way to stockpile breast milk for the workday without having to pump your breasts after every feed.

4. Breast pump

A breast pump is helpful for milk removal for mothers who are separated from their babies, work outside the home, travel without their baby, or wish to pump after a nonproductive feed. There are manual pumps that feature a breast-shield placed over the nipple and areola, squeeze the lever repeatedly, and you pump by hand to express breast milk.

There are battery powered breast pumps and electric breast pumps that power a motorized pump to generate suction. The breast pump flange is attached to the motor by tubing and creates suction to remove milk from your breasts. There are single electric pumps that pump one breast at a time. There are also double electric pumps that bump both breasts at the same time.

5. Pumping bra

A pumping bra is perfect for hands-free breast pumping. If you have a double electric pump, you can place the pump flanges through the bra holes and zip the bra together. It is perfect for the multitasking mama and will hold the pump while you eat, text, work on your computer or play with your children.

6. Breastfeeding bottles

Breastfeeding friendly bottles are perfect for moms who will need someone else to feed their breast milk to your baby. If you plan to introduce a bottle, consider doing it between four and six weeks. There are bottles that are slow flow, soft, and shaped like a breast. These are ideal for babies who have to shift between the breast and the bottle. If it is too easy for baby to remove milk from the bottle, they may drink too much milk.

7. Breastfeeding cover

A breastfeeding cover is merely a suggestion. Some women choose to breastfeed without a cover and some babies refuse to be covered. For those mothers who prefer to be more modest, a breastfeeding cover is a great option. There are nursing shawls, scarves that double as a cover, and a rigid nursing cover. These covers resemble aprons with rigid wire threaded through the top. It pushes the cover out so that a mom can gaze down at her baby during feeds. If you'd rather save money, a receiving blanket will also double as a cover.

8. Breast Milk Storage Bags

Breast milk storage bags are essential for moms who plan to do more than the occasional breast pumping session. These bags store milk in the refrigerator and freezer without taking up much space. After washing your hands, you transfer the milk from the breast pump bottles or milk saver to the bag. Each bag should be labeled carefully and all air removed. If you lay them flat in the freezer to freeze them, you can stack them easily in large plastic bags to maximize freezer space.

9. Breastfeeding Bras

Breastfeeding bras are an ideal accessory for breast pumping or nursing. It is essential that you have a bra that provides support and comfort for your lactating breasts. These bras are designed to allow easy access to the breasts for long-term breastfeeding. Regular bras can interfere with nursing in public. Breastfeeding bras typically unsnap so you can quickly breastfeed and then cover your breasts again. If you opt to use a regular bra, the underwire can put pressure on the ducts and cause a plugged duct or breast infection called mastitis.

10. Breastfeeding Clothing

Breastfeeding clothing, like dresses and nursing tops, are helpful to nursing. Breastfeeding is easier when you can quickly and readily access your breast. The clothing is now very fashionable and comes in a range of pieces. There are dresses, sweaters, dress shirts, tanks, and sweatshirts. Breastfeeding tops and dresses are stylish and can make discrete public breastfeeding easier, but are not absolutely necessary.

11. Lanolin Cream

Lanolin cream provides relief for breastfeeding moms experiencing nipple pain. This cream repairs painful, cracked, blistered, or bleeding nipples. It helps your breasts to heal faster and minimizes any soreness. Apply a pea-sized amount of cream after each feeding to soothe and protect your nipples. The cream is safe for baby and does not have to be washed off before putting your baby back on the breast.

12. Gel Pads

Gel pads are placed in your bra and provide instant cooling relief. They heal sore nipples. The pads are safe, absorbent, and reusable for three days. They come with a fabric backing to minimize friction from rubbing against your clothing.

13. Cold Packs

Cold packs are amazing for mother's breastfeeding with engorged breasts or sore nipples. They are helpful to use after breastfeeding with overfull or painful breasts during weaning or periods of engorgement. You can often place them directly in your bra to keep them secured against the breast. If it is too cold, place a thin cloth (like a baby washcloth) between the breast and cold pack to prevent frostbite.

14. Nipple Everter

Women who have engorged breasts or flat or inverted nipples can use a nipple everter. This is a small, non-invasive tool that provides minimal suction to draw out the nipple. The mother applying the everter determines the strength of suction. They are used to draw out the nipple and give your baby something to grab on to. Once the nipple has been pulled out, baby can easily latch and breastfeed. They come in several sizes to ensure appropriate fit around your nipple.

15. Breast Shells

Breast shells are worn inside the bra. They are lightweight, hollow disks to correct flat or inverted nipples for breastfeeding.

16. Nipple Shield

Nipple shields are useful but should be applied sparingly. It is a short-term solution that should be used under the watchful eye of a location consultant. They are usually initiated in the first days of birth and can be very difficult to wean babies off. A nipple shield is a flexible silicone nipple that a mother places over her nipple during feeding. They are ideal for situations like improving latch with mothers who are engorged, with flat nipples, or infants who are nipple confused.

17. Breast Milk Alcohol Test Strips

Breast milk alcohol test strips are a home test for alcohol in breast milk. You soak the test pad with breast milk and read the results after two minutes. If the color changes at all, it indicates that any alcohol is present in your milk. It detects even low levels. Since there has not been a safe alcohol threshold established, it is unproven what a "safe" amount is. These are a fun party trick but do not have any medical guidelines at this time.

A supplemental feeding system should be used in coordination with a lactation consultant or healthcare professional. It can be used as a way to supplement your baby with breast milk, donor milk, or formula by stimulating your breasts. It is good for mothers with low milk supply or babies with a poor latch. A container of milk is connected to a flexible feeding tube with the other end placed immediately next to mother's nipple. The baby takes mom's nipple and the tube in his mouth when latching. This way the baby has to breastfeed and stimulate the mother's nipples but also gets supplemental milk.

Chapter 25

Bathing Techniques

Being a new parent, you may approach bathing your newborn with trepidation. The good news is that babies do not need a daily bath. Initially, babies only need to be bathed two to three times per week. However, babies have unpredictable bathroom blowouts and spit-up. Some families may discover that your infant needs to bathe more or less frequently.

Newborn skin is different than adult skin and requires specific consideration. Infants are at risk of losing heat quickly through their skin. It is important to keep your infant warm during the bath.

There are many possibilities for bathing your newborn baby. Once your baby can sit in a regular tub, these will no longer need to be a consideration. These first bath options involve:

- A sponge bath
- Small tub bathing basin
- Immersion tub bathing and
- Swaddled Tub Bathing

Some healthcare professionals advise against getting the umbilical stump wet. They encourage you to let the stump fall off between days ten and fourteen before soaking the stump in the bath. However, there are no differences in cord healing for tub-bathed babies when compared to their sponge bathed counterparts.

Tub-bathed babies experienced less temperature loss. They were significantly more content than those who were sponge bathed. Mothers of tub-bathed babies were much happier than the mother of sponge bathed babies. There was no difference in maternal confidence. Tub bathing is a safe and pleasurable alternative to sponge bathing in healthy, term newborns.

A. Sponge Bath

Sponge bathing is when your infant is gently washed with a washcloth over a basin or sink. You carefully wash one part of your baby's body at a time. This is usually the technique that babies are taught in the hospitals. In this technique, it is easy to avoid washing the umbilical cord stump.

The drawbacks of the sponge bath are that it puts infants at risk for increased heat loss leading to cold stress, crying, and agitation. New parents prefer to minimize any emotional distress by their new bundle of joy. This method of bathing can be stressful for parents and babies alike. Because of this, routine sponge bathing is not recommended for ill premature infants

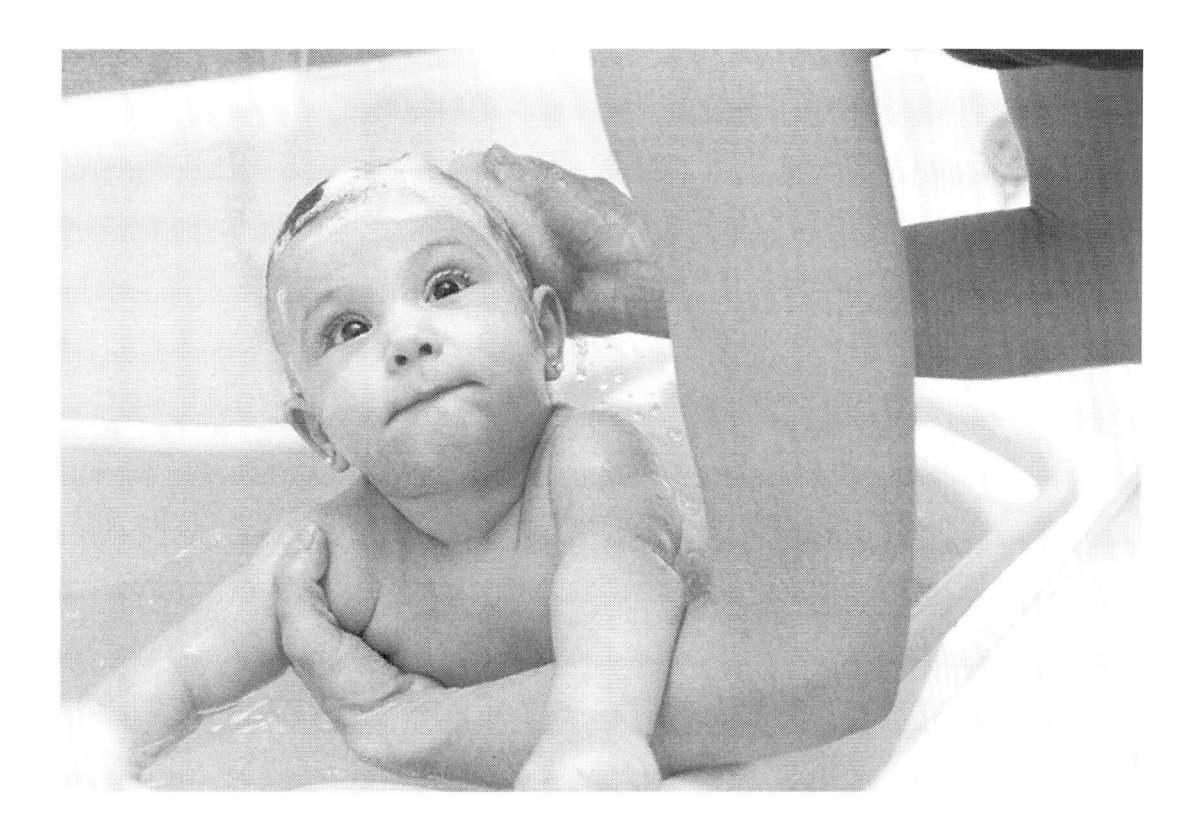

B. Small Tub Bathing

Small tub bathing basins can be used for a bath. The idea is that the infants are too large to fit in the small basin, so their upper bodies are exposed to air. This allows them to bathe in a small bathing container. Babies typically like to be in a small, warm, tight place. The small bathing basin tub essentially cocoons the baby. The tub should use warm water that has been tested on your wrist or inner elbow to ensure temperature adequacy. The drawback of small tub bathing is that it leaves their upper bodies exposed to cooler air and it puts the baby at risk of cold stress

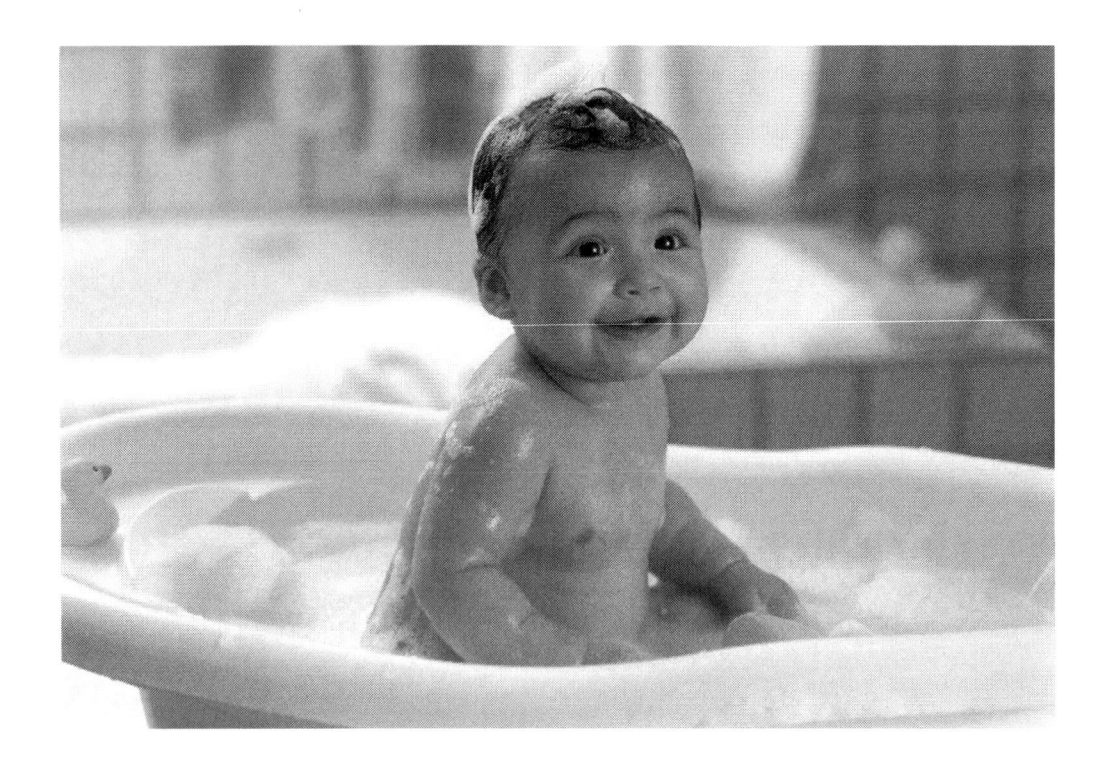

C. Immersion Tub Bathing

Immersion tub bathing is when you submerge the infant's body, with the exception of the head and neck, into warm water (approximately 100.4°F). The bath should be kept to less than five minutes to keep your baby warm and comfortable.

Covering your baby's body with warm water ensures even temperature distribution and minimizes stress to the baby. This means decreased heat loss caused by evaporating water. This bath contributes to keeping your baby warm and the bath enjoyable, which is beneficial for maintaining your baby's temperature and blood sugar. Babies with this type of bath are more content during the bath and their parents report a more serene and pleasurable bath.

Some health care professionals are concerned about the risk of infection and proper healing to the umbilical cord. However, a study found there was no difference in cord healing, bacterial colonization of the cord, or frequency of diaper rash between immersion and sponge bathed infants

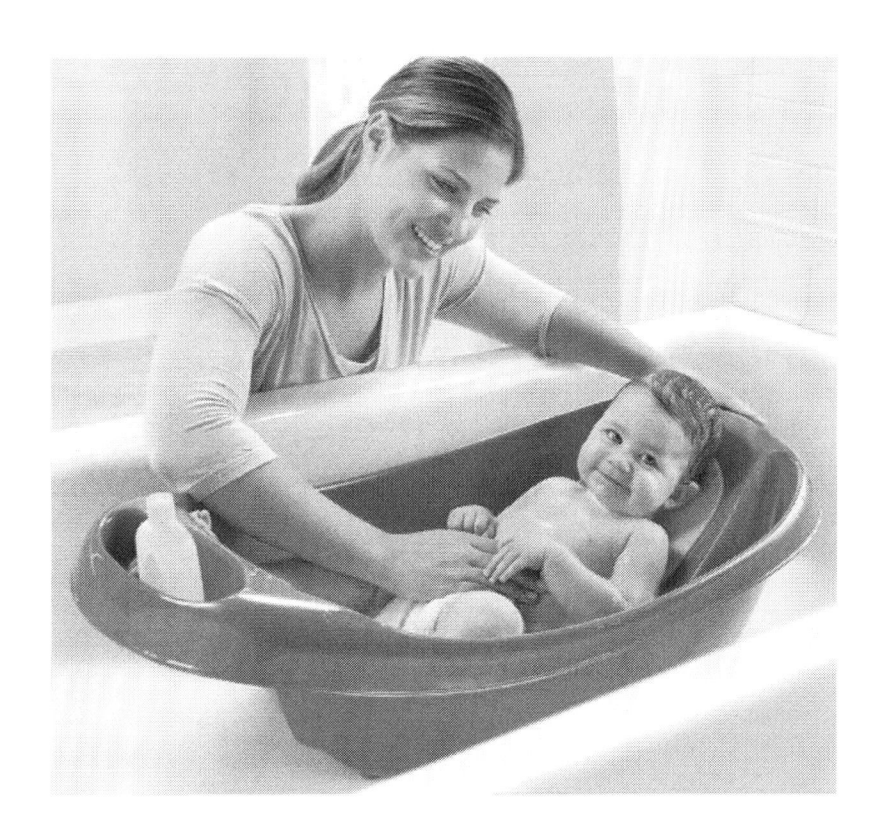

D. Swaddled Tub Bathing

This technique means that infants are swaddled in a soft blanket or towel before they are immersed in a warm tub of water. Swaddling is usually learned from nurses at the hospital. The snug blanket around your baby resembles the mother's womb and is very soothing. When swaddling infants, knees and elbows should be in a flexed position to encourage joint development.

Swaddling your baby decreases random movements of the baby's limbs and promotes a secure feeling. The act of swaddling promotes a calm, quiet state in the newborn. This peaceful bath reduces parental stress and should be initially considered for your baby's benefits.

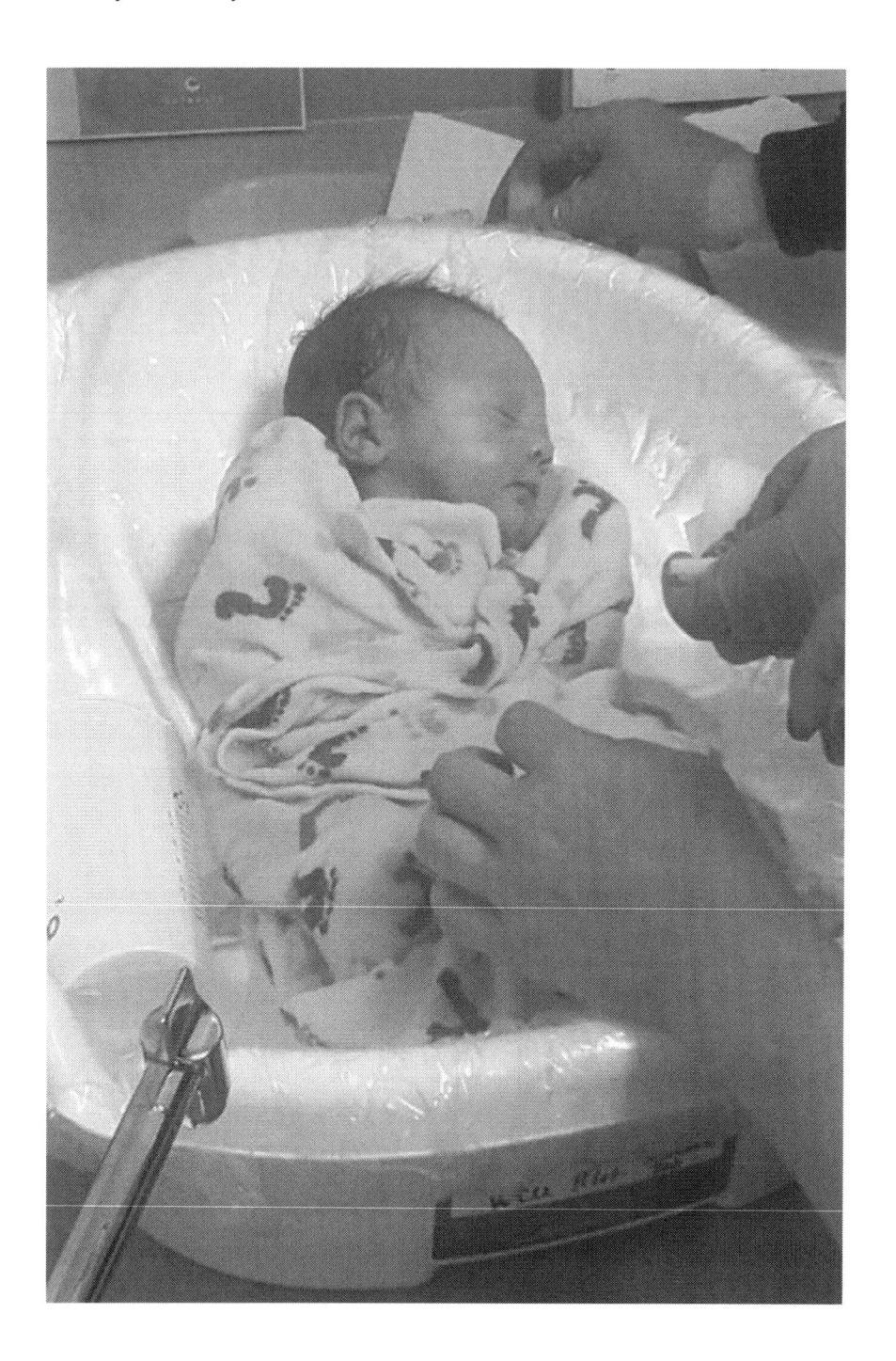

Types of Baby Bathtubs

If you walk into any baby store, you will see a variety of different bathtubs. These bathtubs come in a range of prices and categories. This section will walk through the various types of tubs.

a) The Standard Plastic Baby Bathtub

The standard plastic baby bathtub is a plain tub that sits in your bathtub or on your sink. There is a sloped interior to support your baby, but no bells and whistles. It is usually reasonably priced and an excellent first baby bathtub.

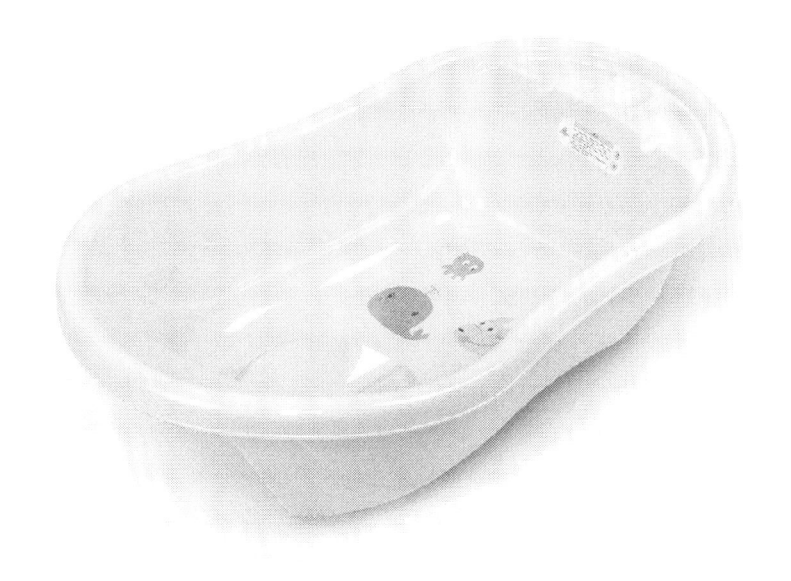

b) The Hammock Baby Bathtub

The hammock baby bathtub will hold your baby in place and support your baby, acting as a third hand so you are able to wash your baby's body. The material cuddles against your baby during the bath. This material acts to calm your baby and enhance your baby's comfort level.

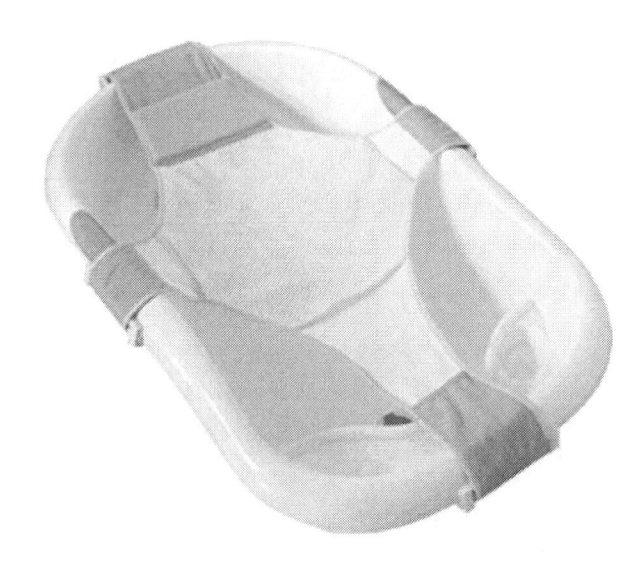

c) The Convertible Bathtub

The convertible bathtub is designed to grow as your baby does. The tub will work from newborn to toddler and give you the maximum value for your money. It can be used in the sink initially, and later gets placed in your larger bathtub.

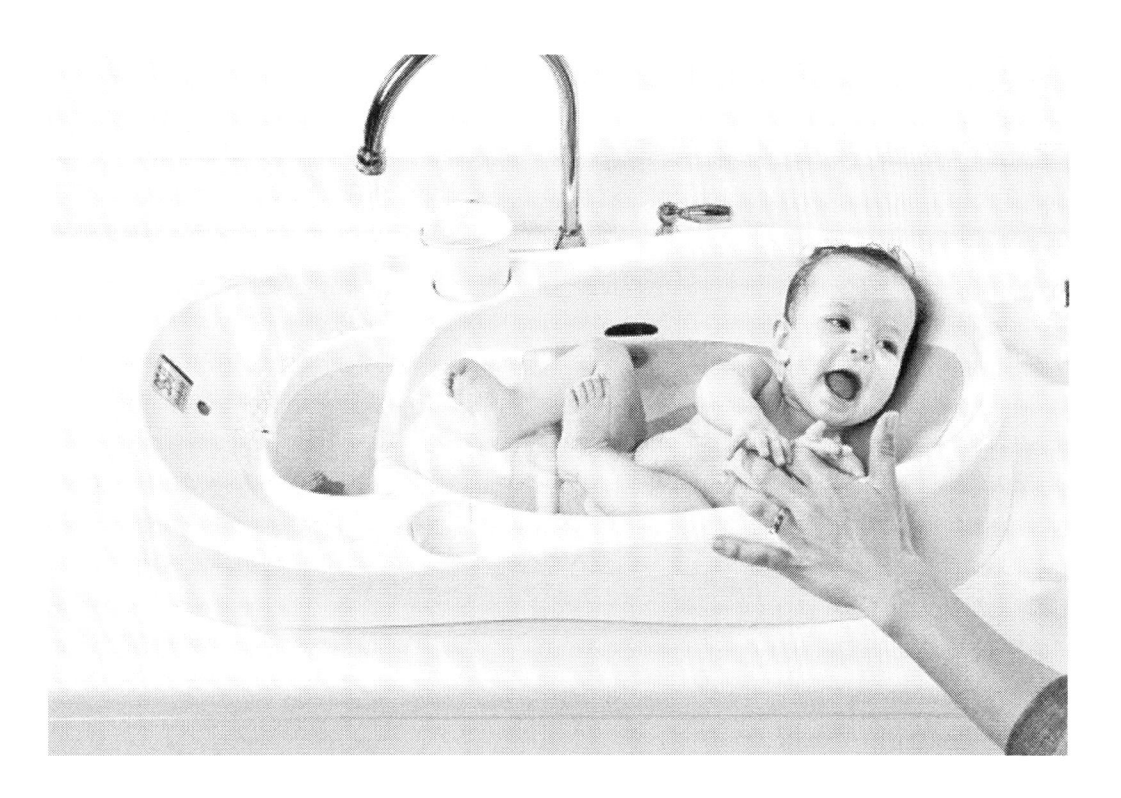

d) The Inflatable Baby Bathtub

The inflatable baby bathtub takes up minimal room. It is fantastic for families who frequently travel or live in small homes without infant bathtub storage space. This tub must be inflated before use. It will hold enough water for your bath and support your baby for an enjoyable bath. The inflatable plastic tub has a nice, soft texture that your baby will not get hurt on.

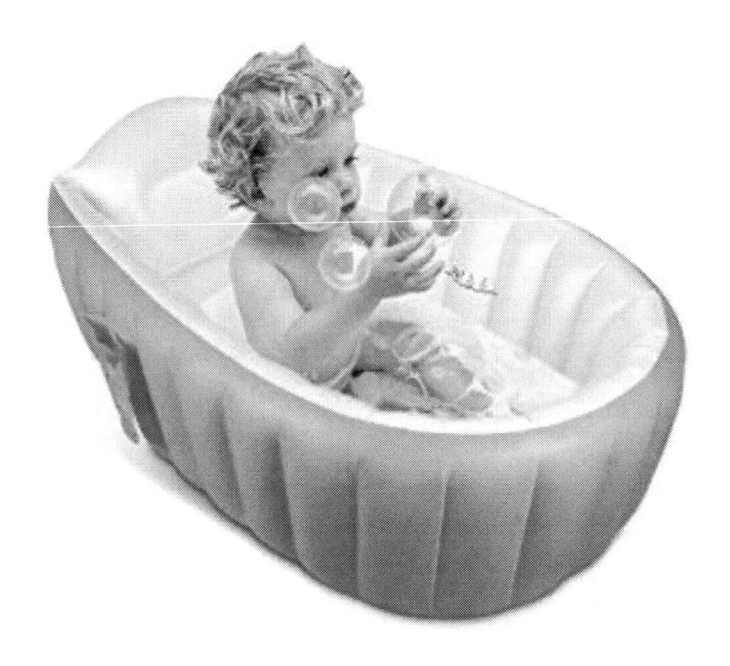

There is a cushion for the bathtub that is an alternative to the traditional bathtub. It does not hold water but supports your baby in the sink or bathtub. You put water in the sink or bathtub, add the baby's cushion, and the water will soak through. However, this spongy material is less durable with less longevity. It usually will require replacement.

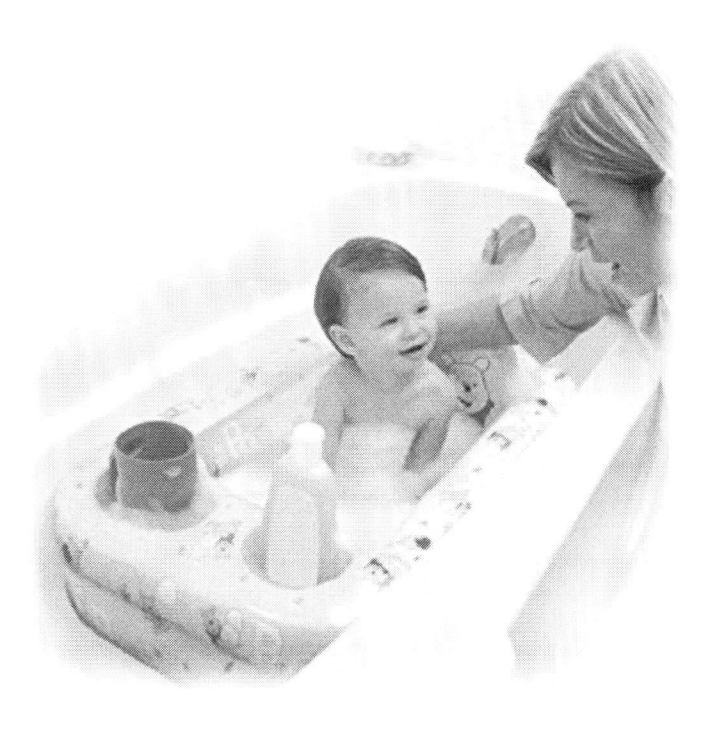

e) Luxury Baby Baths

Luxury baby baths are absolutely frivolous and delightful. They are battery operated with jets, shower nozzles, and bubble machines. They are heavy, inflexible, and not very portable. This is definitely not a required piece of equipment, but occasionally just a fun option.

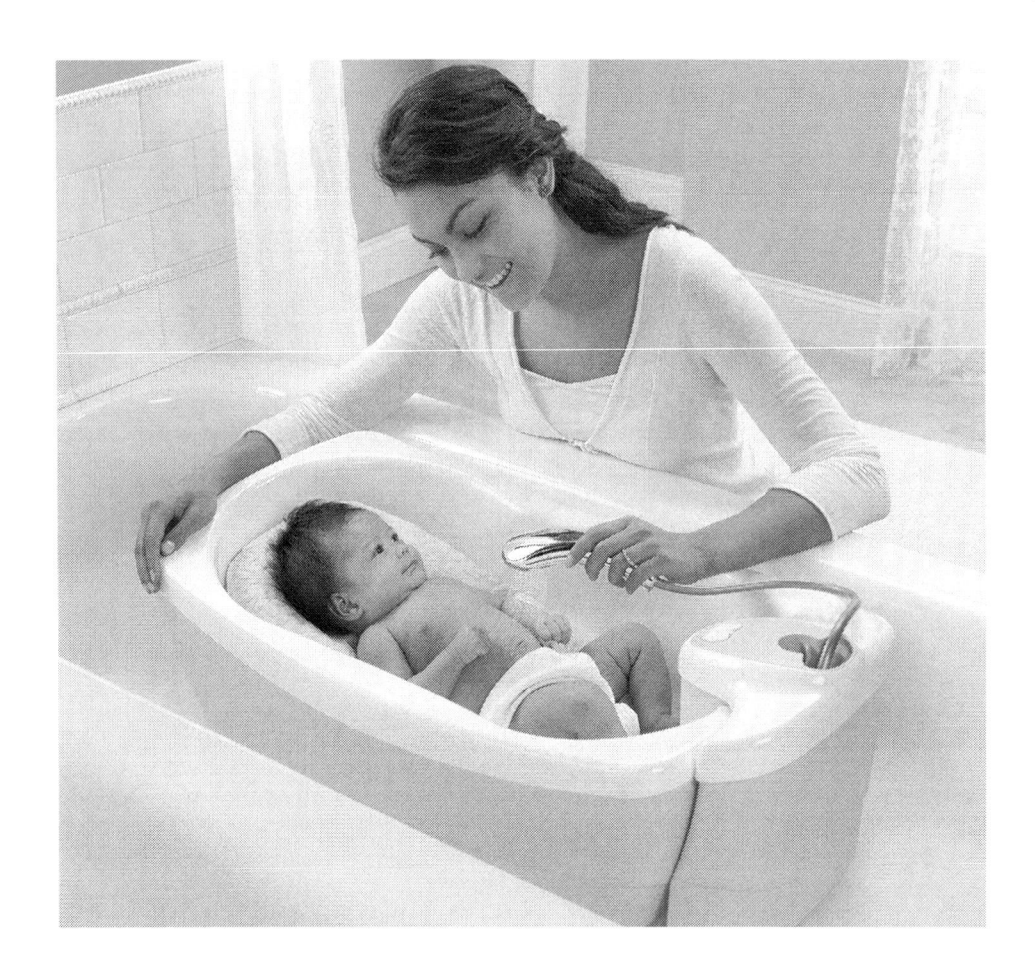

Basic Baby Bathing Tips

1. Delay your baby's first bath.

Delaying your baby's first bath has many benefits. It protects your baby and reduces the risk of infection due to the baby being covered by a thick, white, cheesy substance called vernix caseosa. Vernix contains proteins and old discarded skin cells. It is an essential antibacterial ointment that prevents the transmission of bacteria after birth.

Bathing a baby too soon after birth can be stressful to a baby's system and cause low blood sugar, low body temperature, and promote natural miniaturization of baby's skin. It promotes maternal-infant bonding, increased breastfeeding, and parental involvement because the baby remains with the parents after the birth.

The parents are more involved with the bath, because there are no time restraints and are able to place a higher priority on breastfeeding and bonding. Finally, every hospital worker will wear gloves when caring for an unbathed baby which will decrease the risk of transmission of infections to baby.

2. Babies do not need a bath every day.

Babies only need a bath about two to three times per week. Daily bathing can cause skin irritation. They do not need to be washed from head to toe with soap and only need to be washed when they are dirty. If they are not dirty, warm water is typically enough.

3. Make sure your living space is warm enough for a cold, wet baby.

Set the thermostat to 72 to 75 degrees Fahrenheit. Babies lose heat through their wet skin. Small babies are at risk for getting chilly quickly.

4. Make sure to have all bath supplies ready before starting.

Make sure that you have the bathtub set up in the tub or sink and fill with water. Make sure that you have a cup for rinsing your baby's hair and body, a washcloth, baby wash, and a warm baby bath towel or blanket. Pick a warm room with a flat surface like a bathroom or kitchen counter, changing table, or bed. Cover the surface with a thick towel. Set out a clean diaper and clean clothes. Should you choose to use baby lotion, have that ready.

5. Make the bathtub as safe as possible.

Cover the bath spout with a cushioned cover (or make your own with a washcloth). Line the tub with a soft rubber bath mat. Make sure any glass used in the bathroom (glass doors) is made from safety glass. When your baby gets older, do not allow your toddler to stand in the bathtub. While your baby is an infant, make sure to bathe older children separately from your infant.

6. Do not put your baby in the tub until the water is done filling the bath.

Water that is still running into the tub may fluctuate in temperature. If the water is too hot, it could burn your baby. If the water is too cold, it can cause cold stress. Fill the tub with two to four inches of warm water for babies and no more than waist-high for seated older babies and toddlers.

7. Use a comfortable temperature for the bath water.

Test the water temperature by dabbing your wrist or inner elbow in the water and make sure the temperature is warm, but not too hot or cold. Typically, babies and toddlers prefer a cooler bath than adults do.

8. Do not ever turn your back on your baby or leave your baby alone during a bath.

A baby or toddler can drown in a very small amount of water. Babies have died in less than an inch of water. Some parents stepped away for seconds and it happens very quickly. Do not turn your back on your baby in the bathtub, not even for a second.

9. Avoid causing irritation to your baby's skin.

Avoid bubble baths at any age. Bubble baths put your baby at risk for urinary tract infections. Wash your baby with plain water, always focusing your efforts on the diaper zone and in between chubby skin folds. Be cautious about your selection of soaps and shampoos. Choose a mild, tear-free soap created for babies and toddlers. Babies do not need soap applied on them every bath - it will cause dryness. When used, only apply on the areas that are dirty.

If you let your baby remain in the tub too long, it can cause him or her to get a rash on their delicate skin. If you have an older baby and bath toys, sitting in bubbles can be a prime factor. Let your baby play at the beginning of bath time to prevent their fragile skin in contact with irritating bubbles for too long.

10. Climb into the bathtub and take a bath with your baby.

Take your baby into the bathtub with you. Try to have a support person present to assist with bathing supplies. Make sure that the baby's head is above the water at all times. Having a parent in the bathtub can decrease the baby's fear and promote a calm bath time.

11. If you are a breastfeeding mother, consider nursing during the bath time.

If you are a breastfeeding mother who bathes with their baby, consider nursing while in the bath. This is ideal for couplets that are having any breastfeeding issues. It is also helpful for babies that become distressed during the bath. Nurturing your child with breast milk will calm babies who cry during the bath.

Both moms and babies with breastfeeding issues seem to relax tremendously during this time. There are so many factors at play to promote comfort and feeding. The oxytocin is flowing, the warm water simulates the womb, and they snuggle against your strong heartbeat. This is a great time to attempt latching for babies who struggle to latch or typically require a nipple shield.

Chapter 26

Baby Diapering Methods

For something so simple, the choices and brands for baby diapering are extensive and vary tremendously. The first decision you will need to make regarding baby diapering is between cloth and disposable diapers. If you opt for cloth diapers, you can use either a cloth diaper service to wash your diapers, or you can launder them at home. There are many options for disposable diapers, ranging from traditional disposable diapers, natural or biodegradable.

These types of diapers offer different benefits and disadvantages in the cases of convenience, environmental impact, and cost. Many families have differing views and will make the decision based on what is best for their particular family.

The environmental impact of cloth diapering versus disposable diapers has been evaluated by many studies. A study by Lehrburger and his colleagues found that disposable diapers yield seven times the solid waste when discarded and three times more waste while being manufactured. This is a significant difference in carbon footprint!

The effluents from disposable diapers are considerably more hazardous to the environment than their cloth diaper counterparts. The disposable diapers utilize less water and energy than cloth diapers that are washed at home. Cloth diapers washed at a service use less resources than cloth diapers washed at home. Washing cloth diapers at home uses 20 gallons of daily in a traditional washing machine. This is less if you are using a high-efficiency washing machine.

A. Cloth Diapering

Cloth diapering is good for your baby, the environment, and your pocketbook. It keeps your baby safe from chemical exposure and irritants that are present in disposable diapers.

B. Disposable Diapers

Disposable diapers expose your baby to harmful chemicals. These chemicals can be irritating to your baby's skin and are more likely to cause diaper rash. In fact, disposable diapers contain chemicals called dioxin and Tributyl-tin. Dioxin is listed by the Environmental Protective Agency as a toxic carcinogen. Tributyl-tin has been shown to cause significant hormonal issues in both humans and animals. While studies show that the toxic content in diapers is less than that in our food, it is still best to minimize your baby's exposure to contaminants.

Comparison between both types

a) Cost

Cloth diapering has a large initial start-up investment, but the overall cost savings is significant. The only costs attributed to cloth diapering after the initial purchase is the energy costs for washing and drying and the cost of detergent. One obvious advantage to cloth diaper is the resulting financial savings. You will save more money, the more children that use the diapers that you have purchased. For one child, the cost savings for cloth diapers is $2,000 by potty training.

b) Carbon footprint

The carbon footprint is often an important consideration when choosing between cloth and disposable diapers. There is significantly more energy used in creating and laundering cloth diapers. However, disposable diapers create much more dangerous waste and chemical byproducts.

c) Biodegradability

Disposable diapers take 250 to 500 years to break down in a landfill. Cloth diapers are used repeatedly before eventually heading to a garbage dump. Once there, they take about five months to break down. Cloth diapers can be sold instead to provide a decreased economic impact. This is environmentally savvy and further decreases diapering costs.

d) Washing

The options involve washing cloth diapers at home or using a cloth diaper service. If you use a laundry service, the cost is significantly higher than washing the diapers yourself. However, the carbon footprint is smaller with a laundry service.

Cloth diapers are more time-consuming to change then disposable diapers. Both putting them together to put them on, and preparing them for the laundry takes time. Rinsing, washing and drying the diapers is also slightly more laborious. It only requires an additional two to three loads of laundry per week.

While disposables are typically more convenient then cloth, there are situations where cloth diapers are ideal. For example, you will never have to run out late at night to purchase a package of diapers!

Cloth Diaper Considerations

The cost of cloth diapers can be a large initial cost. It is important to decide how many cloth diapers you will need to purchase. If you are thinking of cloth diapering, this is an excellent addition to your baby shower registry.

Cloth diapering mothers should start with a minimum of a dozen cloth diapers. In order to save money and energy, you should never wash fewer than a dozen. Twenty cloth diapers are ideal to maximize time in between laundering the diapers. If you can afford more, it will make your life easy during the newborn phase. Newborns use ten to twelve diapers per day, babies use eight to ten diapers daily, and toddlers use six to eight diapers.

Some parents decide that they want to use a special diaper pail to place the dirty diapers in to prevent odor and prolong wash time. Changing a cloth diaper in public often requires bringing a receptacle to store it in. The recommendation for a reusable cloth diaper bag is a wet/dry bag.

The ideal bag comes with waterproof lining, a handle or strap, and a separate dry section to zip away separately from the wet diapers. You can use one or two large wet (or wet-dry) bags in the baby's nursery or other areas you frequently change your baby's diaper. You should carry smaller ones for your diaper bag and family car. This type of bag will prevent leaks and odors from escaping. It also will keep dry products away from the wet and dirty diapers.

Wet/dry bags can be repurposed for older children, as well. They make a great bag for swim lessons, the beach, or the pool. Wet towels and swimsuits can be zipped away from the other compartments. You can use one bag to take everything you need for all-day water play.

Some moms choose to use cloth wipes. Cloth wipes can be thrown in the wash with your cloth diapers. They can be bought or made from the flannel material. You can also use baby washcloths, old clothing, or towels cut into small squares. Cloth wipes can be stored dry or wet.

Make sure that your daycare will allow cloth diapers. Daycares that allow cloth diapers often have a preference for the types that they are willing to change. If they are unwilling to change cloth diapers, you may have to switch between disposable diapers at school and cloth diapers at home.

Babies who wear cloth diapers often potty train at a younger age than their counterparts. Babies may be more uncomfortable in cloth diapers than disposables. If your child potty trains quicker, this is a significant saving in cost and economic footprint.

Types of Cloth Diapers

There is an overwhelming variety of cloth diapering choices. These types of diapers vary in convenience, cost, and absorbency. This section will discuss the basic information for each time and recommendations for when they are appropriate.

- **Flats** are a type of cloth diaper that has been used for decades. It is a thin piece of fabric that you can fold in many ways to put on your baby. They are time-consuming and can be folded to customize the absorbency.
- **Pre-fold diapers** are rectangles of fabric that do not require folding. They are already thick in the center to promote absorbency.
- **All-in-One diapers** are the most convenient and similar to disposable diapers. They have a waterproof cover. They come in adjustable or single sizes.

- **Fitted diapers** are similar to an all-in-one diaper, but do not have a waterproof cover built in. The diaper has its own closures and features absorbent fabric that is elastic at the legs and waist for a more "fitted" style.
- **All-in-twos** are similar to pocket diapers and have an outer waterproof cover with an absorbent insert. The difference between pocket diapers is that the insert sits against the baby's skin instead of inside a pocket. These dry faster than all-in-one diapers.
- **Pocket diapers** have a pocket and an outer waterproof cover. The absorbent insert is stuffed inside of the pocket diaper. Pocket diapers come in both single sizes (one size fits all) and adjustable sizes.

Types of Cloth Diapers

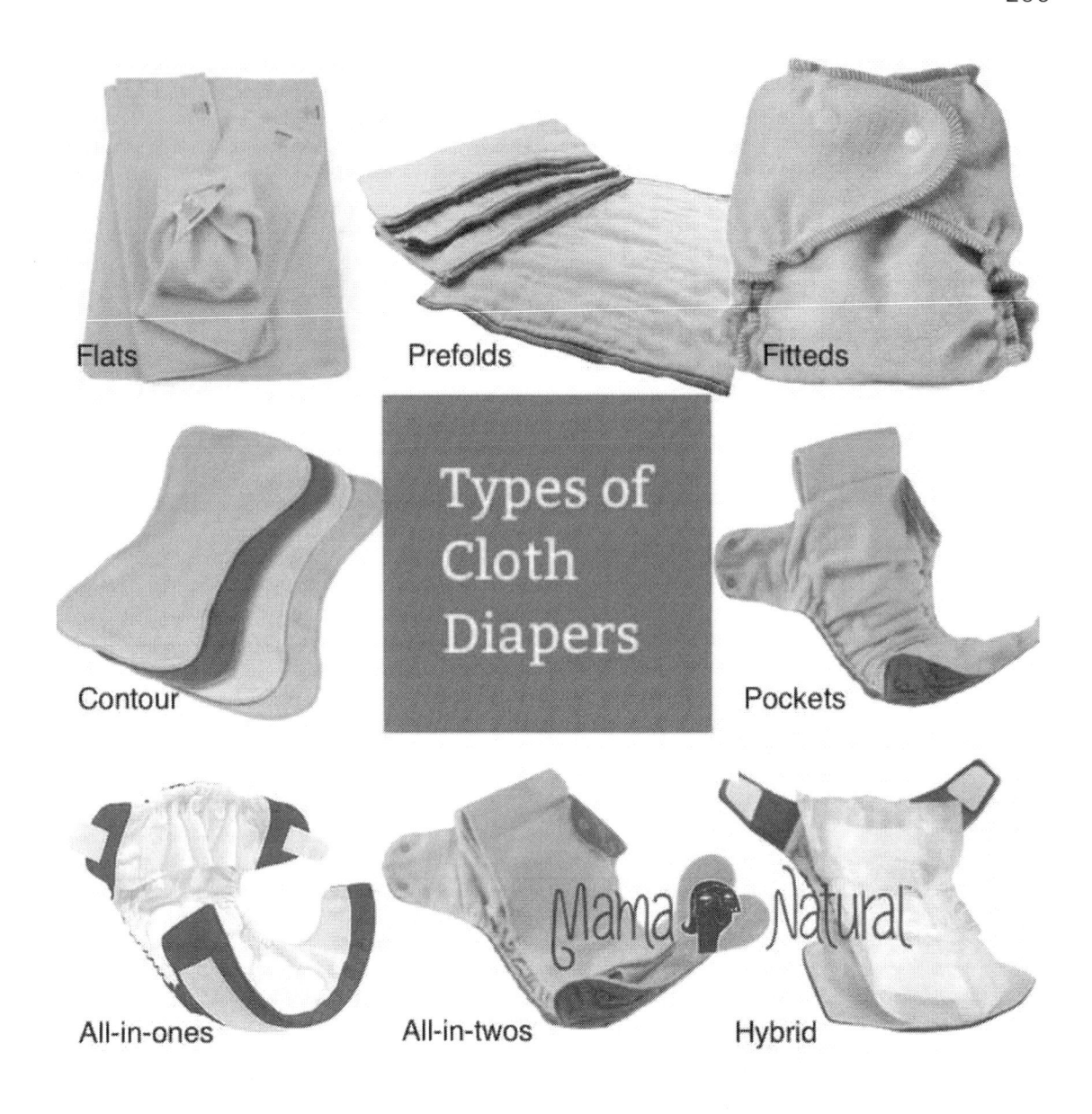

- Flats
- Prefolds
- Fitteds
- Contour
- Pockets
- All-in-ones
- All-in-twos
- Hybrid

The choices can seem overwhelming at first. Even with the wealth of information available about cloth diapering, some families select a few different types to try. However, this can be more costly until you choose the type that works for you. Regardless of what type you choose, this will enable an ideal fit for your family and your baby.

More on Disposable Diapering

Disposable diapers are convenient for diaper changes. They are very portable and cut down on the stress and hassle when compared to their cloth counterparts. Some moms choose to do a combination of both and purchase a small pack of cloth diapers to use at home, and stick to disposable when out and about.

Manufacturing disposable diapers creates a huge economic impact on our planet. Baby diapers contain toxins for the environment. There are diapers available that are responsibly made diapers and biodegradable. However, natural diapers are not chlorine bleached, latex-free, dye-free, fragrance-free and often made of renewable resources like corn. Natural diapers are often more expensive. Some brands have questionable absorbency meaning that they leak and are ill-fitting.

It takes a village to raise a child. Usually, that same village is more comfortable with using disposable diapering. Grandparents, childcare providers, and other family caregivers may prefer disposable diapers. Make sure to discuss diapering preference when lining up care.

Diapering Tips

1. Find a safe place for diaper changes.

Change your baby on a changing pad or table. Make sure you clean off the area to decrease the spread of pathogens. Do not ever leave your baby unattended on a table. Never change a baby where food is consumed or prepared. You want to minimize the risk of infection.

2. Have all supplies ready before starting the diaper change.

Make sure you have a clean diaper, wipes, diaper cream, and the pad prepared before starting.

3. Wash your baby's hands with each diaper change.

Baby's hands need to be cleaned regularly. After a diaper change, you will ensure that you are rinsing off any germs they may have encountered.

For little boys, cover the penis during diaper changes.

The cooler change in temperature can cause infants to let loose. This will help avoid getting showered by your new son.

For little girls, wipe front to back.

This will minimize the risk of spreading germs from her bottom to her urinary tract, causing a painful infection.

What to do in the case of a baby bottom blowout?

Occasionally, newborns have up the back blowouts. You can pull down an infant bodysuit from the neck down over the shoulders. This will prevent you from having to pull a dirty piece of clothing over the baby's head.

Put a clean diaper underneath the dirty one.

This is especially helpful in the middle of the night to catch any stray mess. Sometimes parents change a diaper too early. If the baby is not done, this will prevent you from having to clean up a large mess.

Congratulations!

The fifth character of the password required to unlock the Pregnancy Question & Answer booklet is letter e.

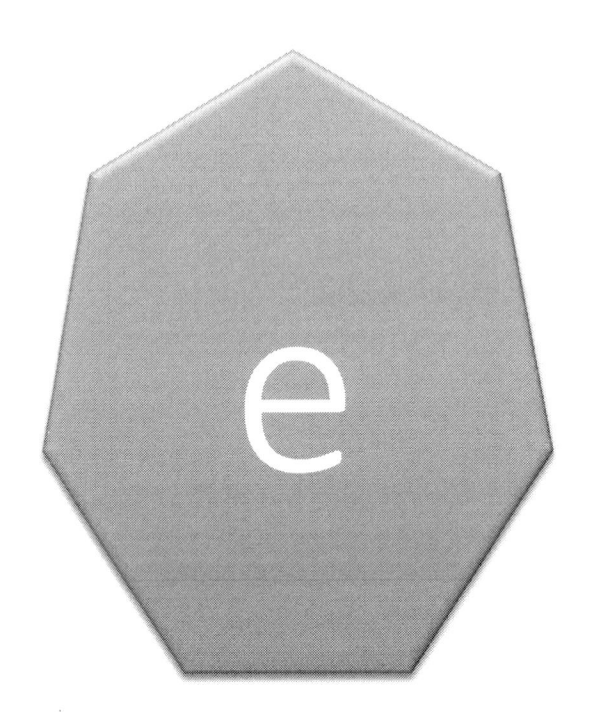

Chapter 27

Baby Circumcision

In the three-decade period from 1979 to 2010, the national rate of newborn male circumcision declined by 10%. According to the Centers for Disease Control and Prevention, this rate decreased from 64.5% in 1979 to 58.3% in 2010.

Newborn babies are born with a foreskin, a piece of skin over the end of their penis. Circumcision is the surgical removal of the foreskin from the tip of the penis. A baby must be medically stable and healthy to have a circumcision performed.

The penis consists of a shaft with a rounded end called the glans separated only by a groove called the sulcus. A continuous layer of skin covers the shaft and glans of the penis. The portion of the skin that covers the glans is called a foreskin.

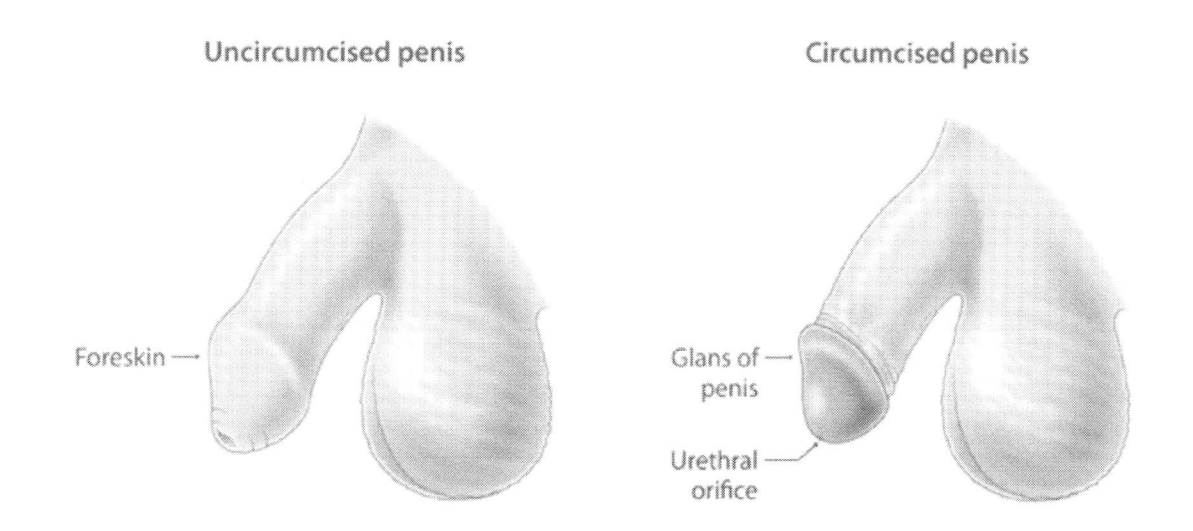

The inner tissue of the foreskin circling the tip of the penis contains erogenous tissue. This means there are nerve endings that provide intact men with the majority of their sexual sensation. Circumcision may reduce sexual sensation.

At birth, urine and feces easily irritate the tender skin on the glans. The foreskin shields the glans from any irritation. However, there are special considerations for hygiene and care of the intact penis.

Care of the intact penis

The foreskin has an inner lining that is a mucous membrane (like what is in your mouth and nose). The foreskin is fused to the glans, which is the top of the penis. As years go by, the inner lining of the mucous membrane will begin to separate from the glans by shedding cells. These skin cells are regularly replaced throughout life.

The discarded cells from the foreskin lining amass as infant smegma, which are whitish, thick curds that move out through the tip of the foreskin. Infant smegma differs from adult smegma.

Specialized glands called Tyson's Glands are located on the glans under the foreskin. They are mostly dormant in childhood. At puberty, these sebaceous glands begin to produce an oily material. This substance mixed with shed skin cells, constitute adult smegma. Adult smegma serves a protective, lubricating function for the glans.

It is not normal for the foreskin to retract easily early in life, but should eventually do so. Typically, it takes until age five to ten years for full separation of the foreskin from the glans to occur. It occasionally happens prior to five years and after puberty. This is normal. Do not forcibly retract the foreskin before it is ready! Once it retracts on its own, the foreskin may then be pushed back, or retracted, from the glans. In younger children, the foreskin may retract spontaneously as children discover their genitals or experience erections.

The intact penis is easy to care for and clean. The infant should be bathed regularly and external genitals washed with soap and water. No special care or manipulation is required and the foreskin should not be retracted. For the first few years, it is only necessary to retract the foreskin if it has naturally retracted on its own. Even then, only an occasional retraction with cleansing beneath is necessary. Once puberty occurs, the male should be taught how to retract the foreskin and clean it daily.

The best advice for hygiene and the intact penis is to let it be. The penis only requires external washing and rinsing. Do not retract the foreskin of an infant, and do not ever force the foreskin back. The natural separation of the foreskin will occur, and at that time the man should move the foreskin back to clean the penis.

The Great Circumcision Debate

The American Academy Pediatrics (AAP) recommends getting male newborns circumcised because of "the health benefits outweigh the risks, but the benefits are not great enough to recommend universal newborn circumcision". The choice to circumcise is best made by the baby's parents along with their pediatrician while considering the best interests of the child. There are many factors to consider involving a baby's circumcision including medical, religious, cultural, and ethnic traditions.

While the procedure is not essential to a child's current well being, there are many medical reasons why a circumcision is done. Men who have been circumcised are less likely to get the human papillomavirus (HPV), human immunodeficiency virus (HIV), penile cancer, prostate cancer, and urinary tract infections. HPV contributes to cervical cancer and other oral cancers. HIV can eventually develop into Acquired Immune Deficiency (AIDs).

The American College of Obstetricians and Gynecologists (ACOG) specifies that circumcision has benefits but the final decision should be left to the patient's parents. Parents may decide against it because it is a painful permanent procedure that is elective. Some parents feel that babies should make that decision about their own body when they are an adult.

It is important to have a skilled professional perform the circumcision. The male circumcision is typically done in a newborn nursery or pediatrician office. Some opt to have it done as a religious ceremony, particularly those who are Orthodox Jewish. The circumcision should only be done by sterile procedure with a professional.

Risks Associated with Circumcision

The complications of male circumcision include a risk of bleeding and infection at the site of the circumcision. There is also the risk of significant scarring on the penis, irritation, and swelling of the glans and inflammation of the urethral meatus (opening of the penis). There is also the risk of injury to the penis and removing too much or too little skin resulting in a surgical revision.

The other drawbacks to expect involve pain and decreased sexual pleasure as compared to the intact penis. However, circumcisions done later in life may be more painful and have more associated complications.

The Circumcision Procedure

The process of newborn male circumcision is a surgical procedure done with sterile equipment. The practitioner opens up the foreskin and examines the glans underneath. Next, the prepuce is separated bluntly from the glans. There are special devices called a Plastibell, Gomco or Morgen clamp used for the procedure. The circumcision device is placed on the penis, and the foreskin is surgically removed. The device remains in place until the bleeding stops.

While many argue that babies do not feel pain, it has been demonstrated that the circumcision causes some pain. This pain may interfere with bonding and behavioral changes. Numbing medication and pain relief are always recommended. Some facilities use a sugar solution during the procedure to minimize the newborn boy's pain. The sugar solution is a 50% dextrose solution. This appears to have no effect on the severe pain of a circumcision. While oral acetaminophen has a small effect on pain reduction after the procedure, the most important aspect of pain relief is the penis nerve block.

There is a dorsal penile nerve block that reduces the baby's pain the most, and the next recommendation is a topical numbing cream. Analgesia should always be used with this procedure. No method of pain relief completely eliminates the pain. Some practitioners opt to give the baby sugar solution during the surgery or oral liquid acetaminophen after the procedure.

After the Circumcision

For the first 24 hours, give the pain reliever called acetaminophen every four to six hours at a dosage of 10 to 15 milligram per kilogram. This means that a six and a half to eight and a half pound baby (three to four kilograms) would get 40 to 60 milligrams of liquid acetaminophen. You should not give your baby more than five doses of acetaminophen in one day.

After the circumcision, you should treat your baby with medication when they are showing signs of pain. These signs and symptoms of pain include fussiness, crying, problems eating, or issues with sleeping. Even though the acetaminophen reduces the baby's pain score, your baby may still experience decreased feeding for the first 24 hours after the circumcision.

Typically, a circumcision is done the day after birth or the next day, as long as the baby is healthy and stable. The recovery after baby circumcision is usually pretty quick. Some babies remain in the hospital for their stay afterward. Some immediately are discharged home.

Postoperatively, you need to check for bleeding and infection. For the first 24 hours, check your son's diaper at every diaper change for active bleeding. The bleeding should be a spot that is smaller than an inch. It is normal to see small drops of blood and skin at the tip of the penis.

Check for swelling of the penis. It should not have significant swelling or drainage with a bad smell. If the baby is fussy and in pain for several hours after the circumcision, that is normal but should not last more than a few days

The diaper changing procedure for a newborn with a circumcision is slightly different. It is important to prevent the penile skin from sticking to the diaper. Apply a topical barrier ointment (petroleum jelly) to the end of the penis during every diaper change and after every bath until the penis is healed.

Female circumcision

Female circumcision is known by a number of names such as cutting, sunna, gudniin, halalays, tahur, megrez, and khitan, among others. It is called female genital mutilation (FGM) by countries and organizations that are opposed to the practice of FGM, like the United States, United Kingdom, and by the WHO.

FGM is the act to intentionally alter and cause long-term injury to the female genital organs. These are done for non-medical reasons with no health benefits to girls and women. The most severe form involves the removal of the clitoris, the genitals, and then the vaginal opening is stitched so that the women cannot have or enjoy sex. A small piece of wood is left to keep an opening for urination and menstrual blood flow. When she is ready to have sex and give birth, the opening must be cut open. Often times, the vaginal opening is sutured closed after finishing their duties to maintain marital fidelity.

It typically occurs to young girls, with a range between infancy and adolescence (newborn to 15-years-old). More than 200 million girls and women across the world currently are circumcised in over 30 countries.

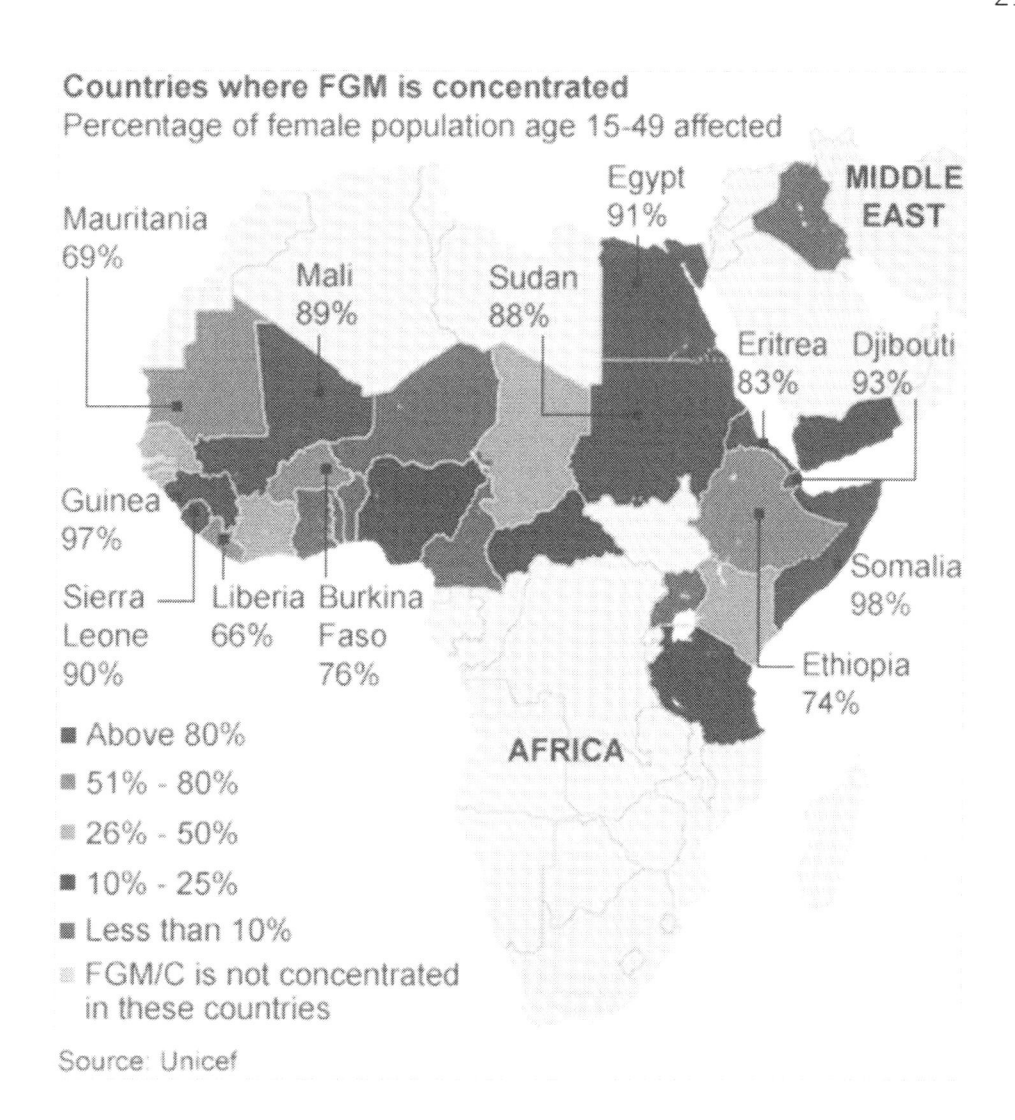

Countries where FGM is concentrated
Percentage of female population age 15-49 affected

- Mauritania 69%
- Mali 89%
- Sudan 88%
- Egypt 91%
- Eritrea 83%
- Djibouti 93%
- Guinea 97%
- Sierra Leone 90%
- Liberia 66%
- Burkina Faso 76%
- Somalia 98%
- Ethiopia 74%
- MIDDLE EAST
- AFRICA

- Above 80%
- 51% - 80%
- 26% - 50%
- 10% - 25%
- Less than 10%
- FGM/C is not concentrated in these countries

Source: Unicef

The major areas practicing FGM include large areas in Africa, Asia, and the Middle East. FGM is also practiced in Eastern Europe, in some communities in Georgia and the Russian Federation. South American countries like Columbia, Ecuador, Panama, and Peru also have significant areas and portions of the population that still participate in female genital mutilation.

Female Genital Mutilation as a Social Norm

Female circumcision is a complicated issue because it is a practice that is deeply entrenched in cultural and social norms in the above countries. Some women see it as their duty for their daughters and feel they will bring shame on their family if it is not done.

In some countries, it increases the marriageability of a young woman. Culturally, it may be considered a requirement of raising a young girl, and the appropriate method to prepare her for marriage.

Female circumcision appears to fulfill the cultural ideals of modesty and femininity. The female genital mutilation preserves the belief that girls are clean and beautiful after removal of body parts that are considered unclean, unfeminine or male.

Many of these countries appear to have strong motivations to continue the traditional practice. There is enormous social pressure to conform to the cultural norm of female circumcision, even it countries where it has been outlawed. Many women have a strong need to be accepted socially and have a fear of being rejected by the community. Worst yet, in some places, FGM is performed on nearly all females and completely unquestioned.

Why FGM is Performed

Practitioners of FGM believe that the surgery will encourage young women to uphold acceptable sexual behavior, ensure premarital virginity, and promote marital fidelity. They believe the practice will reduce a woman's libido and encourage her to resist extramarital sex acts. Some types of the procedure surgically close the vaginal opening so that it physically deters sexual acts.

Female circumcision is not supported by any religious doctrine, however there are some religious influences. Although no religious texts require FGM, many practitioners believe the genital mutilation has a strong religious orientation. Both religious and community leaders take varying position among support or decry its existence.

Women have continued to practice this tradition for their daughters and granddaughters. In a sense, they are now the perpetrators to female genital mutilation. They link it strongly to being socially accepted. Unfortunately, it is a taboo that many do not discuss.

Anatomy of Female genitalia

The clitoris is the sensitive erectile tissue that is small and under the clitoral hood and above the urethra. Prepuce is the fold of skin around the clitoris, also known as the clitoral hood. The labia majora are the outer folds of skin of the vulva, also known as the outer lips. The labia minora are the inner folds of the vulva, also known as the inner lips.

There are four major types of FGM. Unfortunately, with this procedure, anesthetics are typically not used. The most frightening part is that proper surgical equipment may or may not be used. The surgical instruments range from scalpels to knives, scissors, razor blades, or even glass shards. In some cases, girls are held down by other women in the community to complete the procedure.

Type	Name	Procedure
Type I	Clitoridectomy	Partial or total removal of clitoris (In rare cases, only the prepuce)
Type II	Excision	Partial or total removal of the clitoris and labia minora, with or without excision of labia majora
Type III	Infibulation	Reduction of the vaginal opening through cutting and moving labia minora (or majora) through suturing (With or without removal of clitoris)
Type IV	Other non-medical procedures done to genitals	Pricking, piercing, incising, scraping and cauterizing the genitals.

There are a number of problems post-surgically after FGM. The risks include hemorrhage (severe bleeding), vaginal infections, genital tissue swelling, and problems with healing. The associated infections include Tetanus and Bacterial vaginosis. The course of infection ranges from fever, shock, and death. Women who have had FGM are likely to have itching and increased discharge, cysts, and permanent injury to the area. Women may be left with problems urinating and pain with urination (dysuria).

Women with FGM are likely to experience decreased sexual pleasure, sexual dysfunction, and pain during sexual intercourse. Some women who have had Type III FGM must undergo a reversal process called deinfibulation, where the area must be cut open to allow for sexual intercourse and childbirth.

There are complications in childbirth like increased risk of newborn mortality and maternal morbidity. It means mothers who have undergone FGM have babies who are more likely to die. They are also at increased risk of episiotomy, surgical birth, and postpartum hemorrhage. Long-term effects include psychological issues like depression, anxiety, Post-traumatic Stress Disorder (PTSD), low self-esteem and self-worth.

Morality of FGM

Internationally, folks have been working to dissuade practitioners from FGM since the 1970s. It has been outlawed or restricted in many countries. In 2010, the United Nations called upon healthcare providers to stop performing FGM.

Legality of FGM

FGM is Illegal in many places. Unfortunately, it is still performed in many of those same countries. Even in the United States, it has been against the federal law since 1996. The law also prevents vacation cutting, which is the act of removing a girl from the United States to perform FGM elsewhere. Surprisingly, while it is illegal federally, many states do not have a law against FGM.

FGM is Not Illegal in the Following States

N/B: If you can't see all the content in the below table, hold down your thumb on the table and then use the arrow on the left and right side of the table to navigate

Alabama	Hawaii	Kentucky	Montana	North Carolina	Utah
Alaska	Idaho	Maine	Nebraska	Ohio	Vermont
Arkansas	Indiana	Massachusetts	New Hampshire	Pennsylvania	Washington
Connecticut	Iowa	Mississippi	New Mexico	South Carolina	Wyoming

It is illegal for a resident or non-resident of the United Kingdom to perform FGM in or outside of the UK. There is also a law about failing to or protect a girl from FGM that results in 7-14 years in prison.

FGM is also outlawed in Middle East in Kurdish Autonomous Region and a number of African countries. Regrettably, FGM is still carried out in those countries, despite the prohibition against the practice.

African Countries where FGM is Illegal

N/B: If you can't see all the content in the below table, hold down your thumb on the table and then use the arrow on the left and right side of the table to navigate

Benin	Burkinsa Faso	Central African Republic	Chad
Cote d'Ivoire	Dijibouti	Egypt	Eritrea
Ethiopia	Gambia	Ghana	Guinea
Guinea-Bissau	Kenya	Mauritania	Niger
Nigeria	Senegal	South Africa	Sudan
Tanzania	Togo	Uganda	Zambia

Shockingly, it is still allowed in a number of countries. The table shows the countries that have no laws against the practice. Some countries block it from being done at private hospitals, but have no rules against it being done in private homes.

Countries Where FGM is Legal

N/B: If you can't see all the content in the below table, hold down your thumb on the table and then use the arrow to navigate

Africa: Cameroon, Democratic Republic of Congo, Liberia, Mali, Sierra Leone, Somalia

Asia: Indonesia, India, Malaysia, Pakistan, Shri Lanka, Singapore
Middle East: Kuwait, Oman, United Arab Emirates, Yemen, Iraq (central), Iran, State of Palestine, Israel

International Outcry

In the last two decades, there has been a mounting international objection to the practice of female circumcision. The stance of the World Health Organization is that FGM is a violation of the human rights of girls and women. The WHO issued a joint statement against the practice of FGM with the United Nations Children's Fund (UNICEF) and the United Nations Population Fund (UNFPA).

Thanks

Thank you very much for taking the time to read this book. I tried my best to cover as much as I could. If you found it useful please let me know by leaving a review on Amazon! Your support really does make a difference and I read all the reviews personally so I can get your feedback and make this book even better.

If you did not like this book, then please tell me! Email me at drJaneSmart@yahoo.com and let me know what you didn't like or what you wanted to be covered. I continually update my books to cater to my readers needs. In today's world a book doesn't have to be stagnant, it can improve with time and feedback from readers like you.

You can impact this book, and I welcome your feedback. Help make this book better for everyone! Thanks again for your support!

Follow me

To get updates from Amazon whenever I release a new book feel free to follow me by clicking the *orange* follow button (below my picture) on my author page. Clicking on the below picture will take you directly to my author page.

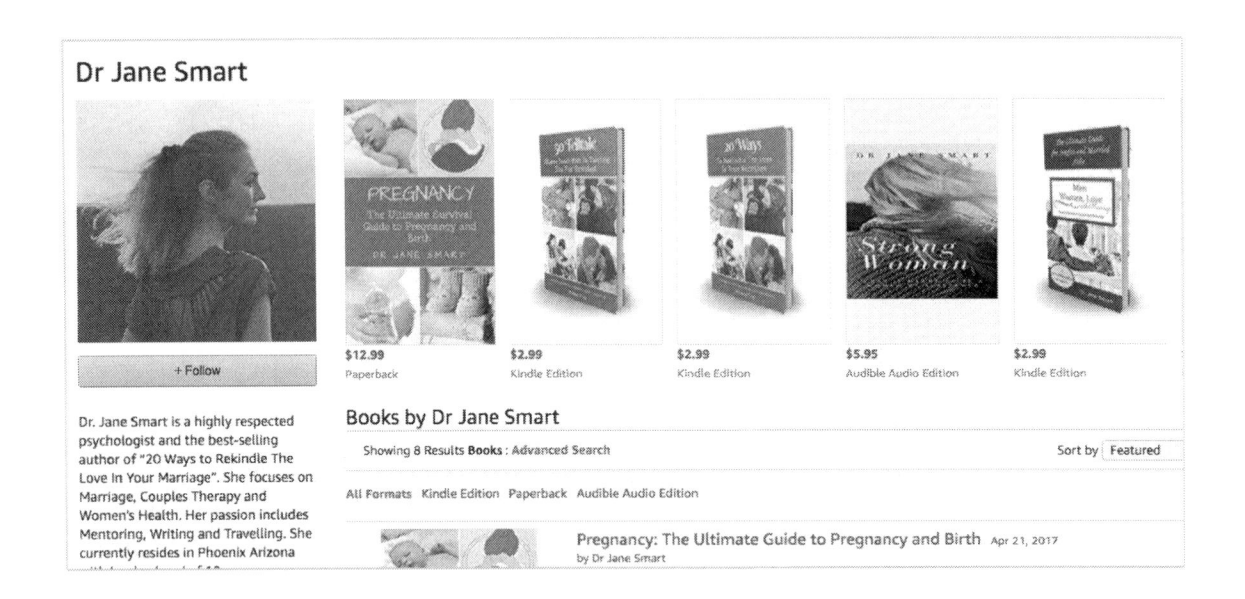

Other Books by Jane

www.MillenniumPublishingLimited.com

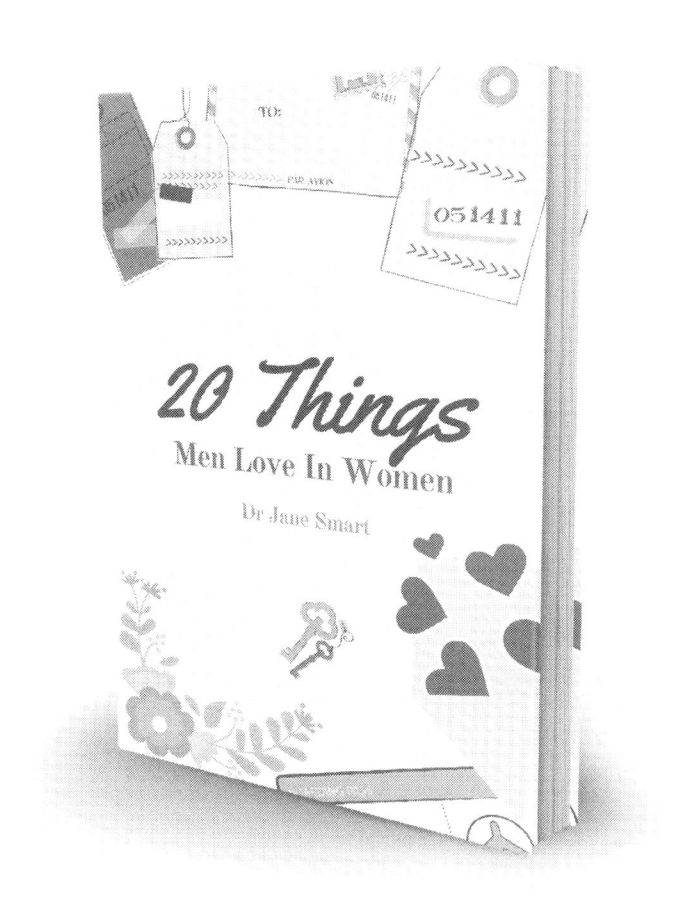

Available in kindle, Paperback and Audio format

*** Buy now for $2.99 (will soon return to $6.99) ***

Get your copy from here www.Amazon.com

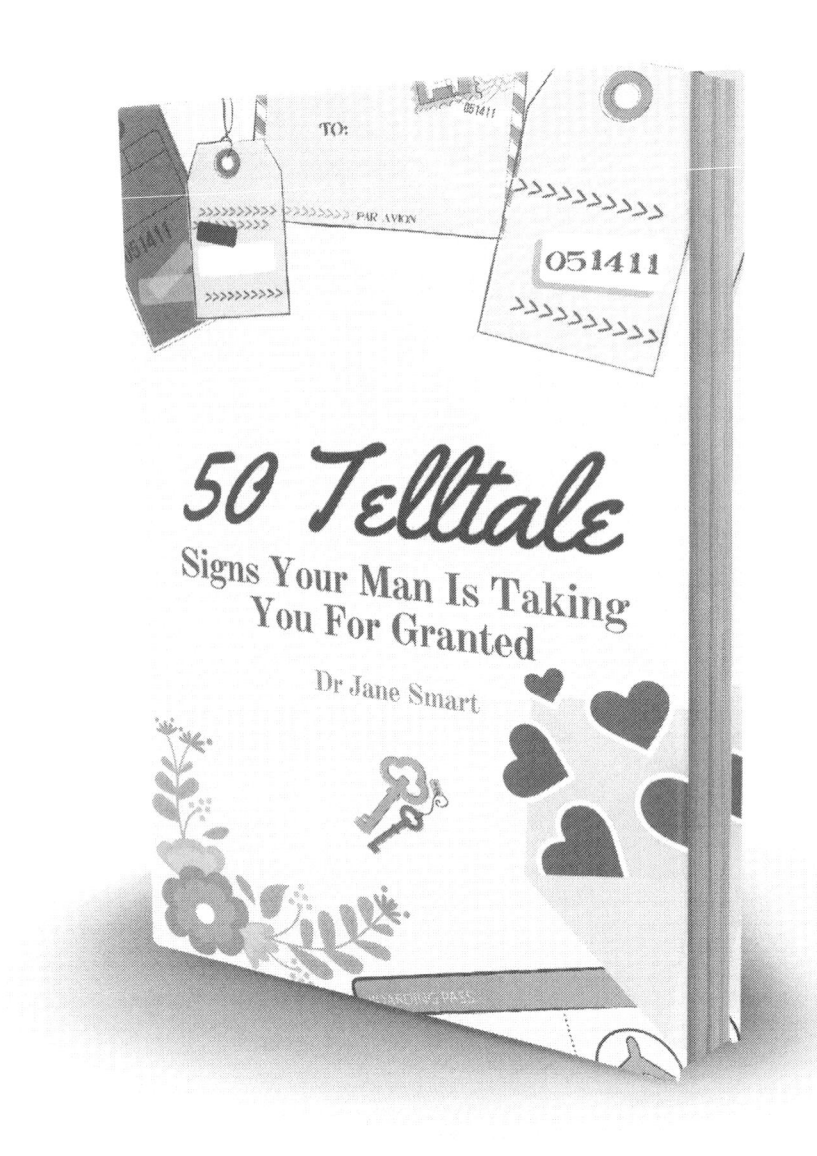

Available in kindle, Paperback and Audio format

*** Buy now for $2.99 (will soon return to $6.99) ***

Get your copy from here www.Amazon.com

Available in kindle, Paperback and Audio format

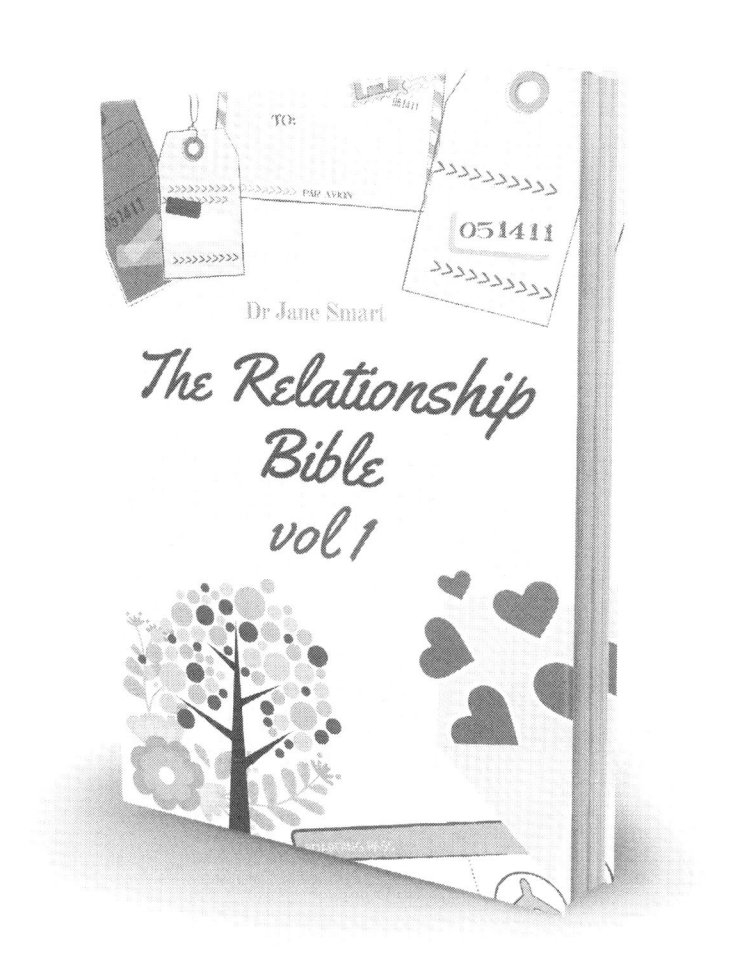

*** Buy now for $2.99 (will soon return to $6.99) ***

Get your copy from here www.Amazon.com

Available in kindle, Paperback and Audio format

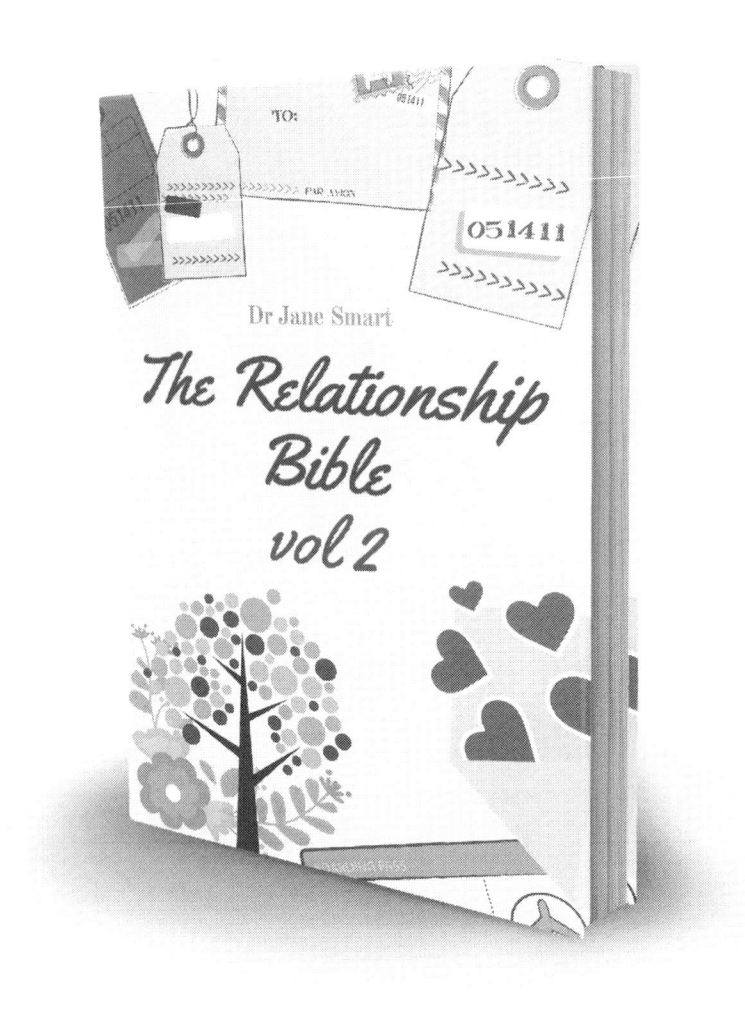

*** Buy now for $2.99 (will soon return to $6.99) ***

Get your copy from here www.Amazon.com

Available in kindle, Paperback and Audio format

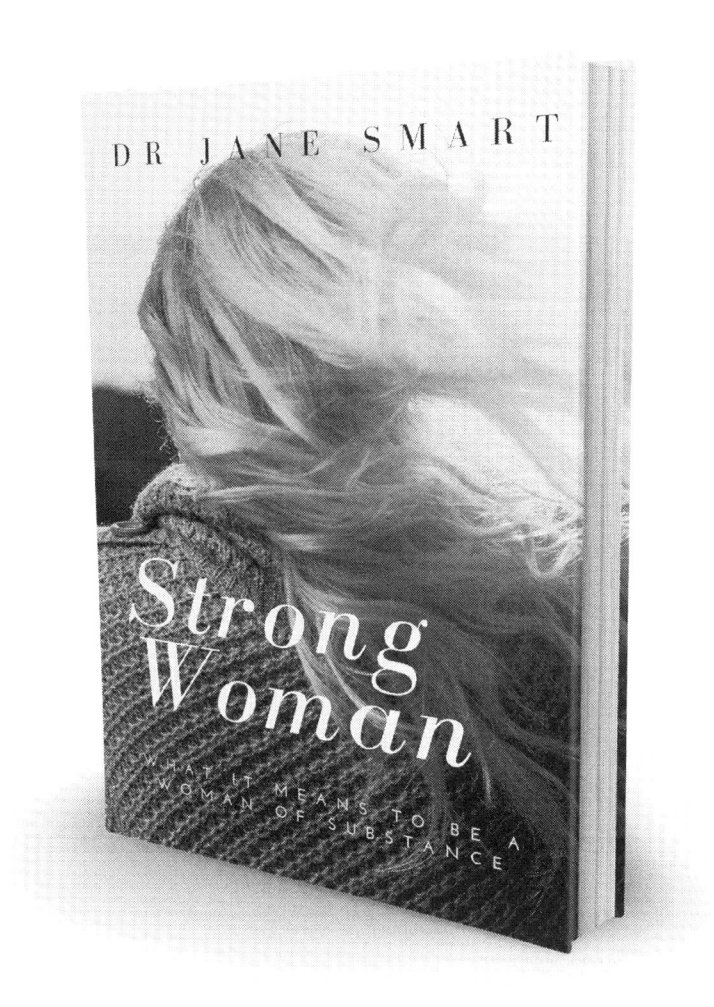

*** Buy now for $2.99 (will soon return to $6.99) ***

Get your copy from here www.Amazon.com

For more quality book, feel free to visit

www.MilleniumPublishingLimited.com

References

American Academy of Pediatrics. (1984). Care of the uncircumcised penis:

- Guidelines for parents (pamphlet). Elk Grove Village, IL: American Academy of Pediatrics.

Lehrburger, C., Jones, C., Mullen, J. (1991). Diapers: Environmental impacts and lifestyle analysis.

Stevens, E. E., Patrick, T. E., & Pickler, R. (2009). A history of infant feeding.

- The Journal of Perinatal Education, 18(2), 32–39. http://doi.org/10.1624/105812409X426314

World Health Organization. (2017). Female genital mutilation: Fact sheet.

Made in the USA
Coppell, TX
03 December 2019